QUARANTINED

QUARA

Dr. Glendenning beginning a head count of detainees, 1917. METCHOSIN SCHOOL MUSEUM

NTINED

LIFE AND DEATH AT WILLIAM HEAD STATION, 1872–1959

Peter Johnson

VICTORIA · VANCOUVER · CALGARY

Heritage House Publishing Company Ltd.
heritagehouse.ca

Library and Archives Canada Cataloguing in Publication

Johnson, Peter Wilton, author
    Quarantined : life and death at William Head station,
1872-1959 / Peter Johnson.

Issued in print and electronic formats.
ISBN 978-1-927527-31-3 (pbk.)—ISBN 978-1-927527-32-0 (epub)—ISBN 978-1-927527-33-7 (pdf)

    1. Quarantine—British Columbia—William Head (Cape)—History. 2. Immigrants—Medical examinations—British Columbia—William Head (Cape). 3. Immigrants—Medical care—British Columbia—William Head (Cape). 4. Public health—British Columbia—William Head (Cape)—History. 5. William Head (B.C. : Cape)—History. I. Title.

RA671.J64 2013   614.4ʾ60971128   C2013-903381-5   C2013-903382-3

Edited by Lara Kordic
Copyedited by Kate Scallion
Proofread by Lesley Cameron
Cover and book design by Jacqui Thomas
Front cover: *Empress of Japan*, Metchosin School Museum (top) and *Disembarking CLC Members on Wharf*, Metchosin School Museum (bottom); back cover: *Chinese Steerage Passengers Carrying Bags*, Metchosin School Museum

 The interior of this book was produced on 30% post-consumer recycled paper, processed chorine free and printed with vegetable-based inks.

Heritage House acknowledges the financial support for its publishing program from the Government of Canada through the Canada Book Fund (CBF), Canada Council for the Arts, and the Province of British Columbia through the British Columbia Arts Council and the Book Publishing Tax Credit.

 Canadian Patrimoine Heritage canadien The Canada Council Le Conseil des Arts for the Arts du Canada 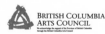 BRITISH COLUMBIA ARTS COUNCIL

17 16 15 14 13   1 2 3 4 5

Printed in Canada

For Leonard, Sonja, and Sofia . . .
may they never be quarantined.

• • •

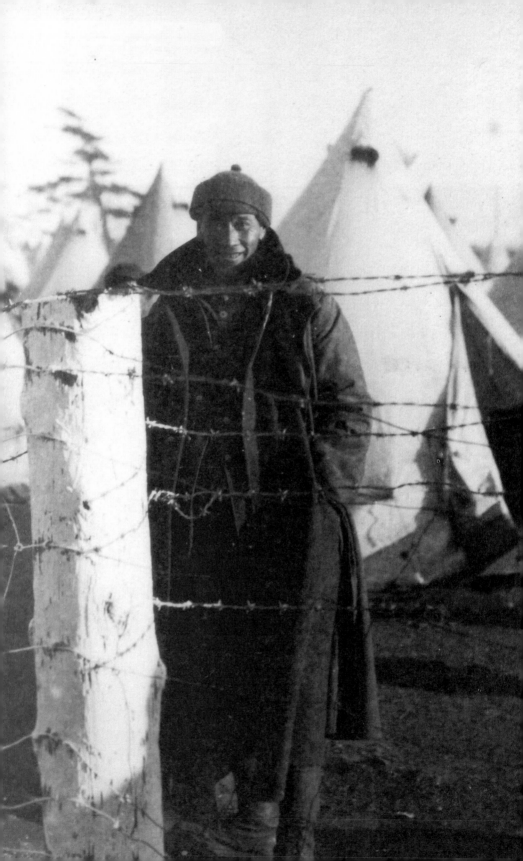

CONTENTS

INTRODUCTION

This is a true story about public health in British Columbia between 1872 and 1959. Specifically, it is a history of a major quarantine station constructed near Victoria at a time when thousands of people were flooding into the province in search of a better life. Up to 1850, this province was one of the last largely unsettled frontiers in British North America. With the discovery of coal near Nanaimo in 1835 and gold on the Fraser River in 1858, it was a place ripe for the taking—and taken it was, from the sea, from the forests, and from the earth itself. By the time the colony of British Columbia joined Confederation in 1871, some forty thousand immigrants had reached these shores. By the time the Canadian Pacific Railway (CPR) was completed in 1885, that number had soared to over 100,000. By the mid-twentieth century, it had reached the millions.

The deluge of immigrants and plunderers did not travel alone. They brought with them the micro-organisms that had been killing millions of Europeans and Asians for centuries. These pathogens threatened whole communities as their carriers weaved new threads into the tapestry of Canadian life. *Quarantined* is the story of the struggle to prevent infectious diseases from entering British Columbia at a time when the infant sciences of immunology and epidemiology were still being challenged by many.

For most British Columbians, the story of the William Head Quarantine Station is completely foreign. Many are surprised to learn that the province even *had* a quarantine station. Yet, in size and significance, it rivalled the quarantine facility at Grosse Île, Quebec, which cleared half a million Irish immigrants in the 1840s while burying five thousand victims of cholera and typhus in its cemetery. William Head was as important as Lawlor's Island

Quarantine Station in Halifax, which examined thousands of Russian Doukhobors and other Europeans until 1938, and it was as influential in Canada as the Ellis Island inspection facility in New York City was in the United States.

In its heyday, the 1920s, the William Head Quarantine Station, some eighteen kilometres southwest of Victoria, encompassed forty-two buildings on a commanding forty-three-hectare headland overlooking the treacherous Race Rocks in the Juan de Fuca Strait. It was built to protect Canada's burgeoning Pacific population from the devastating infectious disease outbreaks that were flourishing on America's west coast and surging in from the Asia Pacific region. It was created in reaction to previous plagues that had laid waste to Vancouver Island's indigenous population in the 1860s and 1870s, and to counter the threat of smallpox among those who chose British Columbia over the poverty, sickness, and oppression of their distant homelands.

By 1925, the detention buildings at the William Head Quarantine Station were capable of holding up to a thousand ship-borne immigrants— two hundred from first and second class, and the rest from steerage. Substantial disinfection buildings housing antiseptic showers washed away most of their surface pathogens, while other large dockside structures held deadly agents like sulphur dioxide and hydrocyanic acid, which fumigated ocean liners such as the *Empress of China* and *Queen Elizabeth*. Huge pressurized steam chambers disinfected clothing and baggage, while the bacteriological laboratory isolated the microscopic agents of smallpox, cholera, meningitis, leprosy, and other deadly contagions. William Head's two hospitals could care for up to fifty patients who arrived in British Columbia at death's door, and its graveyard stood as mute testimony to those who could not be saved.

The reason little is known about the William Head Quarantine Station is that its presence has been kept from public scrutiny. When the quarantine station closed in 1958 thanks to the widely held belief that the battle against infectious diseases had been won, the site became a federally operated minimum-security prison that still operates today. This transformation into a penal institution effectively prevented British Columbia's quarantine story from reaching the general public. Once it became a federal penitentiary, several of the old quarantine buildings were torn down, and the remaining ones were subjected to a series of new practices designed to serve William Head's new corrective function. Those who were keen to investigate William Head's previous life were thwarted. Although many of the old structures remain, access to them is difficult.

Like most other quarantine institutions around the world during its time, the William Head Quarantine Station was organized according to strict lines of social standing; the favours and prerogatives of class and race determined treatment. As such, its civic and federally funded public stance belied a more ominous Janus face—and therein lies the meat of our tale.

• • •

THE STORY OF THE William Head Quarantine Station is fraught with complex meanings. It is a tale of Machiavellian scheming, but also one of the compassion inherent in those who heal. It is a story about community during British Columbia's transformation from wilderness colony into modern state, a time when populations were vulnerable not just to the microbes of deadly contagion but also to the vices of patronage and privilege that often accompanied such cosmopolitan largess. These forces constrained the effectiveness of the William Head Quarantine Station and its predecessor pest houses right from the outset.

At its core, this is the story of those individuals who came here full of hope and were felled by diseases they knew little about. In the end, it is a tale of redemption, about the achievement of science and the triumph of caring. But in the beginning, it is a dark story, a sinister and foreboding tale of political indifference, professional jealousy, prejudice, belief in racial superiority, and rivalries of class. It is a narrative of those who profited from the stricken and those who delivered even more fury and sadness than the microbes that wrought havoc upon already uprooted lives.

All the events in this story actually happened, and all the characters are real. Its sources are annual reports of the chief medical officers at William Head, provincial and federal legislative records, reports of Royal Commissions of inquiry, medical journals, textbooks of epidemiology and infectious diseases, historical texts and papers, photographs, magazines and newspapers of the day, and letters and interviews with old-timers who worked or lived at the William Head Quarantine Station during its early years.

The manner of these sources ranges from scholarly and technical to informal, personal, and passionate. Achieving a balance between them was a knotty problem because several of the incidents and many of the characters described are, indeed, larger than life.

As such, *Quarantined* is partly a clash of the Titans. A once impoverished Scottish laird took on the prime minister of Canada. A former British Army officer and self-proclaimed aristocrat battled with a Supreme Court justice. A past president of the Nova Scotia branch of the Canadian Medical Association destroyed a highly regarded and innovative chief medical officer. Vancouver mayors David Oppenheimer and Frederick Cope played important roles, as did Robert Beaven, mayor of Victoria. Maritime officers Captain H.G. Williams and George Rudlin continually faced danger in conveying the wealthy and the indigent, the well and the sick, to our shores.

The Grand Inquisitors—Judge Begbie, the honourable Henry Pering Pellew Crease, and Chief Justice McCreight—squared off against the pompous ex-military man Major George Bowack. They countered, too, the resentful Dr. Crompton, medical examiner at the William Head Station, and the sycophantic first-class passenger James Ogden Grahame, who both became involved in bloodletting caused by vested interests.

Set against these characters were the real humanitarians, those with compassion who loved the practice of medicine. With them were many others of probity and good faith—doctors Helmcken, Nelson, Watt, Brown, and Jenkins, and nurses Fairweather, Williamson, and Worsley were the healers; Reverend George Hollingsworth Ellison, Canon Bolton, and Reverend Emerson were the faithful; journalists Roy Brown and Altree Coley were honest promoters. Even the Victorian Poet Laureate Alfred Lord Tennyson had a significant part in the William Head drama and in British Columbia's early struggle for a social identity. Those individuals who stood up for the powerless in their forced confinement exemplified the best aspects of our social democracy.

Then there were the stricken, the displaced people who became medical refugees, the ordinary people whose stoic suffering ennobled caregivers to rise far above the tide of human pettiness and act on their behalf. We owe a great deal to longshoreman Harry Farrar, to immigrants Mrs. Bibby and Mrs. Livingstone, to the labourer Joe Wei Chun, and to the night telegraph operator Arthur Monkhouse. We owe much, too, to the lepers Yuen Kow and Lim Bo and to the Russian soldier Abraham Bercovich. We are beholden to Chang Tien Ho (no. 9297) and Lin Chang Cheng (no. 9275) of the Chinese Labour Corps (CLC). And most of all, we owe more than can ever be said to five-year-old Bertha Whitney.

CHAPTER 1 // THE POLITICS OF QUARANTINE

Clinker, you are a most notorious offender.
You stand convicted of sickness, hunger, wretchedness and want.

—Tobias Smollett, *The Expedition of Humphry Clinker*

I can remember as a boy, standing on the deck of the Cunard liner MV *Georgic* as we sailed into New York Harbor. That last day of our voyage across the Atlantic, my older brother and I had a contest to see who would be the first to spot the Empire State Building. He won, so I gave him a thump. No matter, because in that instant when we saw it, we were both transfixed. We were immigrating to Canada along with thousands of other families who fled Britain's economic depression in those awful years before the Beatles. We were en route to Halifax, but my father, who had been a merchant seaman all his life, had travelled the world and he wanted to give his boys a quick look at New York City. I was small and just able to see over the ship's high railing that calm, radiant June morning. Then I saw it, the fabled Statue of Liberty, Libertas, the Roman goddess of freedom with her arm stretched skyward, holding the torch of golden opportunity. My father stood behind us and put his arms around our shoulders. He was a quiet man, a reader who would usher me to the tales of Arthur Ransome, Robert Louis Stevenson, Thomas Hardy, and others. He eagerly read my history books when I went to university.

As we slid past the celebrated monument, he cast a glance at my mother, then recited to us part of its legendary inscription:

. . . Give me your tired, your poor,
Your huddled masses yearning to breathe free,
The wretched refuse of your teeming shore.
Send these, the homeless, tempest-tossed to me,
I lift my lamp beside the golden door![1]

I would be an adult, and my father long gone, before I fully understood the hypocrisy hidden in those words.

"Will we have to go into quarantine, Dad?" I asked, because of my brother. He was pale and thin with pleurisy, and had had poultices and medicine for as long as I could remember.

"No, lad," he reassured me. "Canada has beaten infectious diseases. It's a clean country. They don't have quarantine stations anymore, not since antibiotics."

I remember my mother putting her hand to her mouth and biting the skin around the nail of her middle finger. She was apprehensive, her eyes full of tears. My father's words would prove to be dead wrong.

• • •

IF YOU ARE ASKED to consider the term "quarantine station," think of this image. A father and mother stand beside their two children. They are in a great hall with a huge arched window at one end. Around them are hundreds of other immigrant families. The muted sounds of a thousand conversations bounce off limestone walls. The father is young and bearded. He wears a cloth cap and a worn grey jacket that was once perhaps part of a suit. His pants are baggy and his work boots reveal his status. He is looking up, beyond his family, beyond a sign that he cannot understand to the blue sky streaming in from the great domed window. The mother, looking down, wears a grey cloth coat that is shorter than her cotton dress. Her son sits on the edge of a suitcase, which is tied round with a frayed piece of old rope. He has curly, unkempt hair and wears shorts, heavy socks, and a ragged brown sweater. He is looking at his younger sister, who is absorbed with her doll. She is sitting on top of two worn suitcases that are laid flat on the marble floor.

Although this image conjures up the most famous quarantine stations of them all, the Ellis Island Quarantine Station in New York Harbor, it could be, with some modification, that of a family arriving at the Halifax Quarantine Station, or Grosse Île, Quebec, or hundreds of other stations around the world at the end of the nineteenth century. Consider the reality that Mary Antin suffered when she was quarantined in Hamburg, Germany, for two weeks after fleeing the crumbling autocracy of czarist Russia in 1899. She wrote:

> *Our things were taken away; a man came to inspect us. Strange looking people driving us about like dumb animals; children we could not see crying in a way that suggested horrible things; ourselves driven into a little room where a great pot was boiling on a little stove; our clothes taken off, our bodies rubbed with a slippery substance that might be a bad thing. Suddenly, a shower of warm water let down on us. Without warning we are forced to pick out our clothes from among the others, with the steam blinding us . . . those gendarmes and nurses shouted their commands at us from a distance, as fearful of our touch as if we had been lepers.*[2]

Wherever they were at the time, quarantine stations throughout the world did not engender feelings of warmth.

Now, shift that consciousness forward a century. In 2004—a scant three years after 9/11, two decades after the discovery of AIDS, two years since the outbreak of Severe Acute Respiratory Syndrome (SARS), and amid looming fear of bio-terrorism—the Centers for Disease Control and Prevention in Washington, DC, recommended to Congress that seventeen new quarantine stations be added to the fifty-four still in use in United States territories worldwide. How much have the conditions in these present-day quarantine facilities changed since the days of Ellis Island?

• • •

"QUARANTINE" WAS A LOADED term right from its very beginnings. From the fourteenth to the twenty-first centuries, the well-meaning impulse to impose enforced isolation to prevent the spread of communicable diseases was embedded with politically motivated strategies that reached far beyond the good practices of medicine. It was always the poor, the disenfranchised, and those marginalized ethnic minorities unable to speak for themselves who bore the brunt of tough detention policies rooted more in economics and restrictive immigration practices than in public health.

This Janus face of quarantine began in earnest in the latter half of the fourteenth century. In 1377, the rector of the Republic of Dubrovnik (or Ragusa, which was its Latin name) issued a proclamation called a *trentina*. Ships arriving in Dubrovnik from plague-infected ports were required to anchor in the harbour for thirty days. Soon thirty days' isolation was deemed not long enough to quell the spread of deadly infection, so the rector added ten days to the *trentina* to make a *quaranta*, and the forty-day isolation period, or "quarantine," was born.[3]

Why did the rector choose the forty-day period and not thirty-five or fifty? Answers vary. Dubrovnik was a Catholic city state, and there is speculation that the period was connected with the Catholic observance of Lent, a period of fasting and spiritual cleansing in the forty days immediately before Easter. The thinking went that as the spirit healed, perhaps the body could too. For those who felt that disease was God's punishment, forty days in quarantine was felt to be penance enough.

Another theory suggests that later in the Renaissance, physicians who eagerly dissected the corpses brought to them by the so-called body snatchers became keenly aware of the physical progress of several communicable diseases. Many came to believe that forty days' isolation was the longest period of incubation a disease like the plague might require. Yet merchants believed that a forty-day quarantine period was determined by the cold, hard grip of economics. The trade routes across Asia Minor and Russia to the Mediterranean had to be protected from the plague at all costs. But after forty days, the marketplace would get anxious; prices would fluctuate and speculators could then threaten the stability *and* sovereignty of growing financially independent city states.[4]

Whatever it was, the word "quarantine" stuck. Soon after the rector's decree, the Great Council added separation to the requirement of isolation. The overland traders were isolated in encampments outside the gates of this affluent, walled Christian city. Soon more legislation followed and the police were given powers of enforcement. The following rules—the Rules of Ragusa—were enacted:

- Visitors from states where plague was endemic would not be allowed to enter the city unless quarantined.
- No person from Ragusa would be allowed into the isolation area.
- Those citizens not assigned by the Great Council to care for quarantined persons were not allowed to bring food to isolated people.[5]
- Those in contravention of this law would be fined.

Suddenly, quarantine camps across Europe became seething ghettoes of sectarianism, suffering, and opportunism, with little feeling left for the treatment of infectious disease.

Dubrovnik's laws were important for two reasons: first, they signalled a move away from the medieval idea that disease was a result of God's retribution for human depravity; and second, they demonstrated the degree to which governments would intervene in the lives of its citizens far beyond the claims of public health.

In the fifteenth century, black plague swept along the shipping lanes and overland trade routes from the Middle East to the Mediterranean. Maritime quarantine stations or lazarettos were constructed in Venice in 1403 and in Sardinia in 1450. As quarantined detainees tried to escape the loathsome ghettos, punishment for contravention of quarantine law widened to include the death penalty.

By the seventeenth century, the black plague had spread to Germany, Spain, France, and Britain. When it hit London in 1603, 1625, and 1665, each outbreak killed a quarter of the city's population within months. As epidemiologist Ernest Gilman has written, "in the epidemic of 1603, we have a compelling early-modern forerunner of our own experience of urban plague."[6] Church officials recorded each death, and the results were tallied monthly and published in the London Bills of Mortality. "Searchers" deputized by city authorities had the right to enter suspected houses, report new cases, and effect quarantine legislation. Soon the City of London was sealed off. Schools and theatres were closed and large gatherings prohibited. Businesses considered essential such as greengrocers and apothecaries remained open, but customers had to put their coins in a bowl of vinegar when paying, presumably to sterilize them. Ernest Gilman explains, "Some wore a large, dried toad around one's neck, since it was thought that being a poisonous creature, the toad, even in death would draw the noxious vapours out of the patient's breast and into its own desiccated body."[7] With the germ theory still two hundred years away, alchemy and superstition held sway.

In Germany, the fear of the plague was so palpable that even death proved no escape from the all-powerful arms of quarantine legislation. There is a case on record of a servant girl in Munich who died of the plague in 1640 after breaking a cardinal quarantine order. In consequence, "her body was exhumed, and even while still tied into her coffin, she was hung from a gallows and then burned for all to see."[8] The lesson: Don't mess with the rules!

Since the horrific epidemic of 1348, an estimated 60 million worldwide have succumbed to the plague. In 1665 alone, the plague caused seventy thousand deaths in London. In 1791, Governor Vaudreuil quarantined Quebec City because of it. Traders, sailors, immigrants, and townspeople all knew the telltale symptoms. It began with chills, fever, and swollen lymph glands in the armpits, groin, and neck. Soon, red spots appeared on the skin, the tongue became ghostly white, and the sufferer developed an intense intolerance to light. The inevitable coughing and vomiting of blood confirmed the presence of the pestilence.

Strangely, the role of the rat flea was not known until 1894 when Dr. Alexandre Yersin, who had worked with Louis Pasteur, found that rat fleas, *Ceratophyllus fasciatus,* were abundant on rats in his laboratory in Hong Kong, where an epidemic of plague was raging. Yersin found that the rat fleas were "crowded with the specific bacillus (which came to be known as *Yersinia pestis*)."[9] When the infected fleas regurgitated blood into a human host during feeding, *Yersinia pestis* moved in, either to the lymph nodes or to the lungs. Within the lymphatic system, the nodes swelled as the microbes multiplied exponentially.

When the nodes (buboes) became enlarged and tender, they hemorrhaged, and widespread blood poisoning contaminated the body. When pus-filled buboes exploded, the hemorrhaging caused patches of skin to die. This form of gangrene, known today as disseminated intravascular coagulation (DIC), resulted in large areas of skin turning black, hence the name black plague. Generalized septicemia caused death—a "black death"—usually within seven days.

Since the specific agent of the disease and its progress through the body was not fully understood until the middle of the twentieth century, there was no cure for the plague other than fumigation to kill rats and isolation of infected individuals. Treatment consisted of various ointments and the application of moist towels—essentially palliative care. The deadly little bacillus was safe until the 1940s when streptomycin, tetracycline, and a vaccine were developed.

For over five long centuries, ships and camel trains engaged in commerce from cities such as Hong Kong transported the rats that carried the fleas that carried plague to Sydney, Cape Town, Istanbul, Marseilles, Buenos Aires, Glasgow, London, New York, Montreal, and Quebec.

• • •

IN THE LATE EIGHTEENTH century in Britain, quarantine law and the treatment of infectious disease joined forces to become a powerful means of social control. The English surgeon and essayist John Birch wrote that he opposed universal vaccination on the grounds that "vaccination would eliminate a disease that reduced the least desirable of the population . . . the poor."[10] In his eyes, public health legislation was a convenient way to deal with a growing "troublesome segment of English society."[11]

France also passed quarantine legislation as a means of perpetuating the economic, political, and racial prejudices of the day. The Suez Canal was initially financed by French, British, and Egyptian syndicates, but the khedive of Egypt ultimately went broke and was forced to sell his shares. Britain, under Prime Minister Benjamin Disraeli, snapped up the dividends and made Egypt a loose British protectorate. By 1875, Britain had gained control over the canal. France, desirous to curtail Britain's growing economic authority, built a quarantine station at Port Said, arguing that such a facility would keep Europe free from plagues from the East. But their political objective was different. By demanding that all ships (mostly British from India) be subject to a rigorous and time-consuming inspection, France effectively used health issues to slow down Britain's booming economy.[12]

In America in 1878, an epidemic of yellow fever swept across the Mississippi valley, infecting over 100,000 people and leaving 20,000 dead. As a consequence, "Surgeon General Woodworth sought and acquired greater federal quarantine authority."[13] Through that act, the balance between personal liberty and public health in America was almost lost completely.

In 1884, New York pediatrician Henry Chapin argued that unhealthy vapours called miasmas could cause diphtheria. He wanted to bypass the examination of children's throats in favour of examining the city's sewers. In 1893, he and other medical professionals supported Senator Chandler's quarantine bill, which used the threat of cholera to suspend immigration to America.[14]

In 1892, Dr. William Jenkins, chief officer for the Port of New York, announced that all Eastern-European Jews would be detained before being allowed to enter the city. He had been influenced by the plethora of popular anti-Semitic literature denouncing Jews as "controlling currency, over-throwing government, driving working men into useless strikes . . . and spreading typhus and cholera into the United States."[15]

In 1897, the right-wing Boston lawyer Prescott Farnsworth Hall, secretary of the American Immigration Restriction League, lobbied Washington to disallow Eastern-European immigrants from entering the country. He began with the argument that such contagious diseases as trachoma and favus (a fungal skin rash) were a threat to the American people. Riding on that easily accepted logic, Hall soon revealed his real agenda: he wanted all Eastern-European immigrants with physical disabilities excluded. He even argued that Jewish tailors, who had developed poor postures from being bent over sewing machines all day, were "physical degenerates" and would pass on their deformities to their offspring and ultimately weaken the race. For a time, the United States Senate bought Hall's racial harangues, and by 1907, "several federal immigration acts included these conditions of physical deformity in their medical exclusion categories."[16] Hitler used similar arguments in the 1930s and '40s.

In 1900, a man was found dead in a basement tenement in San Francisco's Chinatown, and an autopsy revealed that he had died of bubonic plague. Panic set in and the city's police began a house-to-house search within the overcrowded community. The search triggered the compilation of a list of so-called unsanitary conditions in an area of San Francisco chockablock with opium dens, herbal establishments, and other strange dwellings.

In 1901, through an executive order, President William McKinley quarantined all Japanese and Chinese persons in San Francisco. Movement to and from their imposed ghetto was prohibited under the widely held assumption that the Chinese were one of the "races liable to the plague." The president's decree was finally challenged and overturned as it was found to be in violation of the equal protection guarantees afforded by the Fourteenth Amendment of the US Constitution (1868).[17]

From 1917 to 1919, more than 300,000 American soldiers were diagnosed with venereal diseases acquired largely from prostitutes. Several states passed legislation that resulted in VD-infected prostitutes being incarcerated in quarantine. Kansas further criminalized prostitution so that guilty men and women were quarantined alongside common criminals. "Fewer men ended up being incarcerated largely because VD was viewed primarily as a female affliction."[18] The law remained on the books until 1956.

In British Columbia, "on April 1, 1882, a leprous Chinaman was hanged and partially burned by his countrymen in New Westminster, in order to prevent contagion."[19] In April 1892, when a Chinese passenger from the *Empress of Japan* was found to have smallpox, Caucasian passengers were simply moved on to Vancouver while more than five hundred Chinese in steerage were quarantined in tents at the Albert Head Quarantine Station. At the height of the ensuing epidemic, Vancouver City Council provided a "pest house" solely for the Chinese on Deadman's Island in Coal Harbour.[20]

Later that same year, smallpox took the lives of three people in Calgary's close-knit Chinese community; a carrier of smallpox was tracked to his dwelling in a Chinese laundry. In spite of the fact that four Chinese were found to be entirely smallpox free after the required period of quarantine, a mob of three hundred non-Chinese Canadians ransacked the community while police constables simply stood by.[21]

Tuberculosis was the cancer of the nineteenth century. It consumed millions of emaciated victims who coughed themselves to an early grave. It targeted the underclass and gained prominence as it mushroomed among the urban poor of Europe, as the unemployed migrated from city to city. TB thrives in an oxygen-rich environment; the bacterium, once inhaled, moves to the lungs. Houses in nineteenth-century Europe, as in other parts of the world, were taxed partly on their number of windows, so profit-minded landlords simply bricked over existing openings or built structures with fewer windows. As penurious bohemians were crowded into the damp, small rooms full of exhaled air, the disease naturally raged.[22]

The phenomenal spread of tuberculosis in Russian and American prisons in the twentieth century exemplifies how quarantine legislation was used to contain criminals as much as disease. In the Siberian gulags of the early twentieth century, "the rates of tuberculosis were some 40 to 50 percent higher than they were in surrounding areas."[23] Although tuberculosis was said to be almost non-existent in Russia by 1960, when the USSR collapsed in 1991, the state released thousands of TB-infected prisoners into a vulnerable population. In the absence of a social safety net, TB's incidence once again soared.

The collapse of Russia's public health system surely expedited the country's tuberculosis problem, but that collapse was the result of the "corruption, criminalization, and piratization of the Russian government and its assets."[24] Without the strong arm of Soviet Communism, it was no longer possible to administer expensive TB drugs to an increasingly drug-resistant general population. The marginalized, the malnourished, the homeless, and those forced into crime were doomed. What officials did not seem to get is that Western drug companies keep the cost of new medication inordinately high and MDR-TB (multi-drug-resistant tuberculosis) readily escapes over prison walls.

In America, the situation is worse. The US has the highest per capita rate of imprisonment in the world, with a large surge in drug-related convictions occurring in the 1980s during the Reagan administration's war on drug-related offences. Between 1980 and 1990, the number of people incarcerated for drug-related offences increased from 10,000 to 100,000. As the prisons filled, they became little more than human warehouses where tuberculosis raged. TB rates jumped more than 150 percent in that ten-year period. According to Paul Farmer in his book *Pathologies of Power,* the war on drugs was "used as a ruse for managing inequality and criminalizing poverty. [It] became a war on individual drug users and petty traffickers, rather than those who finance or run the drug industry." As in Canada's penal detention of aboriginals, "by 1995, 7 percent of all African-American males were interned."[25]

In 1991, Rikers Island jail in New York City revealed the highest rates of MDR-TB in the country (500 cases per 100,000 people), and when its spread to wardens, visitors, and surrounding communities was clearly identified, alarm bells began to ring. "Multi-drug-resistant tuberculosis tied such institutions together in a vast chain, conveying the mutant strains rapidly across the nation," Farmer asserts.[26] The courts eventually stepped in and demanded caps on the number of inmates.

Canada's "get tough" Omnibus Crime Bill passed in 2012. With double-bunking in prisons being offered while more prisons are constructed under the mantra of cost-effective measures, drug companies remain free to set prices. Large numbers of Canada's Aboriginals and others face the prospect of tuberculosis as a form of punishment. The misadventure continues.

In 1986, the Cuban Ministry of Health invested over 3 million dollars to begin widespread testing of groups considered to be at high risk for human immunodeficiency virus (HIV). By 1993, over 12 million tests had been carried out. Those testing positive were detained in newly built quarantine stations and interrogated about their past travel and sexual history. Cuba's enforced quarantine policy was lifted in 1994, but as of 2003, over half of those detained still remained in government sanitoriums.[27]

Quarantine has its benefits, but it also has its risks. As pathogens become increasingly resistant to drug treatment, our only choice is to employ restrictive measures of disease control. While quarantine legislation in the beginning attempted to protect healthy populations from infected minorities, history has shown us that it has been used by those desirous of social control. The establishment of a quarantine station on Canada's west coast was grounded in a humanitarian impulse to protect the citizens of British Columbia from infectious diseases, but it, too, suffered from the politics of privilege, the economics of indifference, and the stigma of racial profiling.

CHAPTER 2 // BERTHA WHITNEY AND THE HOUSE OF DEATH

A recent edition of the London [medical journal] Scalpel states that either smallpox or scarlet fever will absolutely disappear in twelve hours if the following remedy be used: Sulphate of Zinc, one grain; fox-glove (digitalis), one grain; sugar, half a teaspoon. Mix together with two teaspoons of water. Dose: Take a teaspoonful every hour; smaller doses for children according to age.

—*The British Colonist*, June 14, 1872

Little Bertha Whitney was just five years old when she arrived in Victoria on June 13, 1872. Bertha was bright-eyed, good natured and bubbling with curiosity, and her parents adored her completely. Already terrified by a string of smallpox epidemics that had swept through their hometown of San Francisco that spring, they scraped together what little money they had and fled California in a hurry with their precious darling. Victoria, British Columbia, seemed safe. On June 6, 1872, with Bertha enveloped in her father's arms, they boarded the steamship *Prince Alfred* at San Francisco's Hyde Street Pier. In that short walk across the gangplank, the Whitneys' life and the state of infectious disease control in western Canada changed irrevocably. Bertha's sickness and the events surrounding her short life were decisive in British Columbia's pursuit of a federal quarantine station on Canada's west coast. What began as a simple act, taken in good faith to sidestep a fearsome pestilence, soon became a bizarre morality play whose themes of money, race, and class would haunt BC's efforts to maintain that station for the next eighty-five years.

Bertha seemed as spirited as ever when they left, but that soon changed. Dense, cold, wet fog held the wheezing, worn-out steamer off Point Lobos, California, for eight hours. The delay did not really matter, because the 160-foot *Prince Alfred* had never been known for its dependability or speed. It was built in 1852 in one of the many shipyards on the River Wear estuary near Sunderland, England, specifically for Australian immigration and trade, but the ship soon failed in that venture because it could not compete with larger and faster ships. The *Prince Alfred* languished under Grenadian registration until 1871, when it was bought by Rosenfeld & Birmingham of San Francisco to begin a heavily subsidized mail service between that city and Victoria. Some makeshift cosmetics added more cabin and steerage space for extra revenue, but even then the old steamer wasn't up to its task. It was underpowered, its condensers unable to maintain a constant head of steam, prone to breaking down, and susceptible to rolling in any running sea. Yet the one thing that the *Prince Alfred* still had at that juncture was cheap fares—and for the anxious Whitneys, cheap fares were good enough.

It was raining when the *Prince Alfred* left San Francisco that Monday morning. Once outside the bay, it ran smack into a series of heavy southwest gales that would last for the next seven days. By the third day outbound, little Bertha Whitney had become nauseated and developed a fever. Captain H.G. Williams presumed it to be smallpox; with seventy-four other passengers on board, he had good reason to worry. On June 11, off Cape Foulweather, the captain had the cabin adjoining the Whitneys' vacated, and her parents were instructed not to mingle with the other passengers.

Still two days from Victoria, Captain Williams saw Bertha's condition deteriorate, and ordered a steward, normally detailed to first class, to attend to her exclusively. Finally, at 3:00 p.m. on Thursday, June 13, seven and a half days after limping out of San Francisco Bay, the old steamer dropped anchor in Royal Roads in the Juan de Fuca Strait opposite Esquimalt Lagoon. Captain Williams immediately ordered the yellow flag of quarantine to be raised to the top of the foremast and fired two guns to announce to those on shore the gravity of his plight.

Nothing happened.

• • •

NOTHING MUCH HAD BEEN happening for quite some time. Early explorers knew that epidemics of smallpox had struck local Native populations long before Fort Victoria was even established. Peter Puget, Captain George Vancouver's second lieutenant on the *Discovery*, noted in his May 1792 log that he had seen Natives in a canoe in the Gulf of Georgia in which "two or three had lost an eye and were very much pitted with the smallpox."[1] By 1853, ten years after Camosack had become Fort Victoria, smallpox struck again. Little was done except to isolate the few contagious white merchants according to the Hudson's Bay Company (HBC) policy. They had caught the disease from Native traders.

On March 18, 1862, the side-paddle steamer *Brother Jonathan* arrived in Victoria carrying a white miner from San Francisco who was hoping to cash in, albeit belatedly, on the Fraser River gold rush. He arrived with an active case of smallpox. A week later, on March 26, the *British Colonist* reported another case had arrived with the steamer *Oregon*.

For all of its dreaded history in Europe, the prevailing attitude toward smallpox among white Europeans in Victoria at the time was one of nervous confusion. The *British Colonist* sounded the ominous note: "The cases may be few, but they are dangerous, and as the harbouring of such a disease is to injure this place, we must stop people from coming here."[2] It was not to be.

Smallpox is one of the most virulent of all infectious diseases. It had, by the end of the nineteenth century, killed or disfigured untold millions of people in Western Europe. It was estimated that smallpox killed half a million people in each of the epidemics of the 1820s and 1840s in Germany and France. In Britain, overcrowded embarkation cities such as London and Liverpool had smallpox mortality rates that were a quarter of the birth rate. In China, the disease had been laying waste to millions since the twelfth century.

One particular early treatment had been known for years. As the disease spread throughout the body, it erupted in pockmarks on the skin. Pus taken from the mounds of someone who had survived a mild case of the disease was scraped onto a small darning needle and scratched into the upper arm of a person hoping to beat the disease. Though this practice, called variolation, had been practised in Africa and Asia for many centuries, it was rife with devastating complications ranging from hepatitis to deadly septicemia.

Edward Jenner started developing a vaccine for smallpox in the 1790s from less dangerous cowpox particles. In 1796, he perfected his vaccine, but anti-vaccinationists loudly disclaimed its use until the very end of the nineteenth century. The causative agent, a large virus of the *Poxviridae* family, was not isolated until the 1950s.

In Bertha Whitney's time, the morphology and transmission of smallpox was only just beginning to be understood. Today it is well known. Viral particles enter the body through the upper respiratory tract after face-to-face contact with airborne droplets from an infected person. The virus then multiplies in the warm, moist lymph nodes and enters the bloodstream, where after four or five days, it invades the epidermis causing telltale red marks on the skin. Just prior to their eruption, the patient suffers fever, general malaise, headache, prostration, back and limb pain, and vomiting. After three to five days, small red, flat areas (macules) in the dermis swell into elevated lesions (papules) and become infected. This infection then explodes onto the skin. But the papules also extend deeply into the dermis, causing great pain. Concentrated on the face, forearms, wrists, palms, and soles of the feet, the pustules soon turn into recognizable disfiguring scars. After a week, scabs develop over the scars and result in permanent pockmarks. Other bacteria, such as staphylococci, often contaminate the pustules and cause even more serious complications such as abscesses, septic joints, osteomyelitis, and corneal ulcers (which often resulted in blindness). An ointment was used around the eyes to ease itching, but it did nothing to prevent the general toxemia, septic shock, and ultimate demise of most patients suffering from advanced forms of the disease.

Yet for all this, Victoria's predominantly British citizens were still confused over the threat of smallpox in their city. There had been relatively few instances of the disease among white settlers in the colony prior to Confederation, and the British felt that with a bit of caution and their self-proclaimed God-given superiority, they would keep it so. The new germ theory, still vigorously challenged by many, had yet to moderate this view; however, racially based fears had a greater impact.

"Imagine for a moment what a fearful calamity it would be, were the horde of Indians in the outskirts of town, to take the disease," wrote the *British Colonist.* "Their filthy habits would only perpetuate the disease."[3]

It has been estimated that over three thousand First Nations people and some disillusioned miners were camped within shouting distance of Fort Victoria in the early 1860s. Onlookers described the conglomeration of tents and shanties as an ongoing party of drinking, slave trading, fighting, and whoring. Sure enough, smallpox swept through the encampment like a grassfire. By early April 1862, a visiting missionary to the Songhees Reserve near Ogden Point found half of the seventy inhabitants dying. Two weeks later, twenty Aboriginals, acutely susceptible to the disease, were dead. When HBC physician Dr. Helmcken learned of the Songhees Reserve outbreak, Governor Douglas prompted him to vaccinate thirty Natives. By May 1862, he had vaccinated five hundred more. As the precious vaccine ran out, panic set in.

Governor Douglas knew full well that many Natives were considered an affront to the sensibilities of British colonists living in Victoria. To many, they were simply an eyesore living on the streets, hanging about in shop doorways, and filling the pit of the local theatre. Yet Douglas also knew the value of Aboriginals to the burgeoning local economy and therefore considered them worth protecting. Fearing that smallpox would inevitably leap from infected Natives to susceptible, unvaccinated Europeans, Douglas also needed to conserve what little vaccine he had left. He acted quickly. Those living on the Songhees Reserve near the old fort were given eviction notices. Soon after, Douglas ordered their encampment burned to the ground.

The governor believed that the ensuing Native dispersion was the fastest way to mitigate the spread of the disease among Victoria's unvaccinated white population. The reality was the devastating spread of the epidemic among Aboriginals up Vancouver Island. In May, it had crossed to Fort Simpson. By June, the Native populations of Nanaimo and Cape Mudge were dying in scores. Before the epidemic was over, smallpox would kill more than twenty thousand Natives, a third of the Aboriginal population of Vancouver Island.

As it spread farther up the coast, terrified Aboriginals and settlers alike turned to helping themselves. They had heard of the European measure of variolation and eagerly sought completely untested variations of the procedure. Britain had banned variolation with smallpox excreta in 1840 in favour of Jenner's safer vaccine, but the law had lapsed in its colonies, including Canada. It wasn't long before a black market of "scab vaccine" was peddled up and down the west coast. According to Douglas Hamilton, "Scabs were collected from smallpox victims, dried for several days and hawked for two-bits apiece."[4] Sniffed as powder, swallowed, or ground and dissolved and inoculated directly into the arm, smallpox, septicemia, and other deadly contagions scudded north.

While the humanitarian city fathers did construct two temporary smallpox isolation huts in Victoria, one for the whites and one for Natives, newspaper magnate Amor De Cosmos made his feelings known about the Aboriginal facility. "The hospital, so called," he wrote, "is only a place where the victims may die in a heap without being obnoxious to anyone."[5] Others stepped up and challenged the existing indifference. Anglican bishop George Hills sent two missionaries north to vaccinate terrified Natives. "He was," the *British Colonist* reported, "anxious to furnish the means requisite for this purpose from the very liberal donations made in England toward the British Columbia Indian Mission fund."[6] His motivations, at least, were clear.

Then, like the mercurial flight of a flock of birds, it was over. In Victoria, things quickly returned to normal by July 1862. "Smallpox seems to have exhausted itself,"[7] the *British Colonist* stated smugly, "and no fear of its spreading among the white population is entertained."[8] In August, a small outbreak flared up among some Natives living in the ravine behind Johnson Street, and deaths among Natives were still being reported in Cowichan Bay until December; these incidents were not considered serious.

Overall, the white population had been spared. The 1862 epidemic had been an unwelcome and unnerving aside, yet for most of the "British Raj" on southern Vancouver Island, it *was* just an aside. Many believed that birthright, racial isolation, and a higher standard of living among the English in their fair city had left them largely untouched.

And other than the establishment of the Victoria Board of Health, the whole subject of the provision of a proper quarantine facility for the west coast, or the introduction of a quarantine protocol for inbound ships, was virtually ignored. It would remain so for the next ten years.

Indeed, none of the early immigrant voyages to Victoria were ever cleared through any quarantine facility, even though the ravages of infectious diseases in Europe were well known. When the sailing ship *Silistria* arrived in November 1862, nearly half of its three hundred steerage passengers, mostly young English labourers, were put to work within days of arrival, building roads in Metchosin or clearing Governor Douglas's land in Fairfield. No one thought to interview the ship's officers about shipboard diseases—not that it would have done much good in this instance because *Silistria*'s so-called doctor hated his job, kept no records, and spent most of his time during the voyage dead drunk.[9]

When the *Robert Lowe*, a sail-assisted steamship from London, dropped anchor off Victoria on January 10, 1863, after 116 days at sea, it carried a precious cargo of 36 marriageable young women slated to wed single men on the frontier. Two of the girls developed highly contagious tuberculosis en route. They were whisked away to the Royal Navy hospital in Esquimalt, where they died two days later. The rest came ashore just hours after landing with only a cursory, dismissive examination.

In 1868, another small outbreak of smallpox struck Victoria and claimed fifty Natives. This time, however, five local white settlers also succumbed. With these European deaths, the reality of infectious diseases carried by thousands of shipboard immigrants arriving on Pacific shores was brought home. But it wasn't until the arrival of the *Prince Alfred* that windy afternoon in 1872 that this lingering anxiety, not to mention a libellous responsibility, forced reluctant lawmakers of Victoria to take decisive action to halt incoming contagion once and for all.

• • •

ALL NIGHT LONG AS Bertha Whitney's condition continued to worsen, *Prince Alfred* lay on its chains. Anyone on shore looking seaward in the crisp morning westerly would have readily seen see its yellow quarantine flag snapping in the clear, azure sky. Yet no one acknowledged the ship's predicament. All afternoon that Thursday, a frustrated Captain Williams and several increasingly angry passengers kept a vigil for any sign of shore-side movement. There was nothing.

Finally, around noon on Friday, June 14, some twenty-four hours after the *Prince Alfred* first anchored, an exasperated Captain Williams lowered a longboat and he and Mr. Webster, the Wells Fargo & Company agent on board, rowed for shore. Captain Williams was determined to alert civic officials of the status of his ship and the increasing seriousness of Bertha's sickness. Mr. Webster was more concerned with the dispatch of the all-important Victoria-bound mail, and as he climbed into the dinghy he nimbly placed a small sack containing an assortment of letters—likely infected—under his seat. The captain never spied the bag until the longboat reached the dock. Once it was discovered, Williams explained the oversight to the postmaster in town and offered to row the mail immediately back out to his ship. The postmaster accepted the captain's explanation but felt his offer was entirely unnecessary. The letters and whatever they carried remained on shore.

It took over an hour for Captain Williams to find Dr. Matthews, Victoria's newly appointed health officer. When he finally was located, the doctor's profanity loudly revealed his wrath. Before he followed Captain Williams out to his ship, Dr. Matthews secured the presence of a hastily inducted, plain-clothed security officer, Mr. Peter Eddy, to enforce the so-called Dominion quarantine regulations. The delay, Dr. Matthews would announce later, was due to the fact that the *Prince Alfred* was "supposed to have anchored in Victoria Harbour"[10] and not some miles away in Royal Roads, something that Captain Williams may not have known. Besides, Matthews added, "I did not hear the guns, but followed [the ship's movements] as quickly as possible as the rough weather permitted."[11] From the shore in Esquimalt, Matthews also asserted, "there was no yellow flag flying."[12]

Twenty-six hours after the arrival of the *Prince Alfred*, a physician and an ardent neophyte official were finally seen heading toward the stricken ship. Dr. Matthews wrote later that once he was aboard, he advised Captain Williams to secure a quarantine flag from Captain Cator of HMS *Scout*, which was anchored nearby.

In the meantime, many passengers on the *Prince Alfred* were incensed by the lack of medical attention. Many more had grown frightened by the delay, and a few resorted to violence. Dr. Matthews reported that "from the moment of my arrival on board, I was subject to more insults than could be uttered by any animal in the shape of man."[13] The *British Colonist* was kinder and remained within the bounds of Victorian decorum, noting that "when the Health Officer went aboard, he was received with marked evidence of disfavor from the passengers who groaned and hissed at him."[14]

Matthews immediately ordered two men whom he believed to have smallpox to be taken ashore. He suspected too that little Bertha Whitney might have the disease and that her condition warranted special attention. When he left the ship without her, several passengers saw this as callous disregard for the little girl's plight, and they erupted in rage. The morning newspapers noted, "Matthews was struck with potatoes."[15]

As Dr. Matthews left, Officer Peter Eddy remained the sole guardian of quarantine regulations on board. He had to deal with an enraged Captain Williams, who was fuming over Matthews's allegation that he had not observed proper signal procedure. As a coastal ship on a regular service from a smallpox-infected city, the *Prince Alfred* would have had the full complement of signalling flags on board, including the yellow flag of quarantine. It was outrageous for Captain Williams to be charged with not flying the quarantine pennant when he had been preoccupied with Bertha Whitney's condition for the whole voyage. Had Dr. Matthews pointed the finger at Captain Williams to deflect his own inattention and delay?

Soon, Captain Williams became suspicious over the presence of the lone "security" officer on board. Claiming that Peter Eddy's papers were not official, he demanded that the *Prince Alfred* be allowed to take on fresh water as its tanks were quickly running dry. Resolute and officious in his superior's absence, Officer Eddy stood his ground. He refused to allow the ship to move, insisting that no one was to leave or come aboard.

Dr. Matthews had departed the *Prince Alfred* to relate conditions on board to the Victoria City Council and seek their instructions. All that Friday evening, June 14, Mayor Lewis and his councillors wrestled with the destiny of those on the ship. Its arrival had already garnered some bad press, and Mayor Lewis knew that if he did not act with dispatch, events might explode in his face. He was facing the mass detention of a goodly number of quarantined passengers who also happened to be Victoria's rich and well connected. Besides having extensive political clout, they lived in a city with virtually no facilities for any extensive quarantine confinement. But Lewis knew that a sick child was a threat to the whole community and that she too required isolation. He also understood that many of Victoria's upper crust would not take kindly to the special treatment of a destitute American family and their steerage acquaintances. Beyond this, Mayor Lewis eyeballed the potentially staggering expense of a large-scale quarantine detention facility, and the even more sensitive issue of who would have to pay for it. To add insult to injury, those first-class passengers Mayor Lewis sought to help were left helpless on a godforsaken ship with "not a drop of something to drink."[16]

Early in the morning of Saturday, June 15, Victoria City Council supported Mayor Lewis's plan. He would act irrespective of provincial or federal government obligations, and he would act with resolve—the others be damned. With advice from Attorney General John Foster McCreight, Mayor Lewis chose to spend whatever it cost to stem the disease in his midst. He would seek financial compensation later.

Later that day, Dr. Matthews returned to the ship and told Captain Williams that the *Prince Alfred* was now formally under quarantine. He also gave him an official letter confirming that Mr. Eddy was indeed "sworn in as a special police officer."[17] Given the need for water, Dr. Matthews gave permission for the ship's boats to secure fresh water from Royal Navy ships anchored nearby, provided the boat's crew had no contact with anyone else. However, when Williams lowered a longboat to do just that, Captain Cator of HMS *Scout* refused to let a quarantined vessel approach *any* of Her Majesty's ships. Trying to calm the outrage, Dr. Matthews told the passengers that Bertha Whitney would be removed and those passengers and crew who had had contact with Bertha's parents or their steward would be quarantined ashore. The ship, he said, would be fumigated in the course of time. He then stated that only a few officers and a skeleton crew were to remain on board.

When the affected first-class passengers learned that their steward had literally rubbed shoulders with Bertha's parents, they realized that they were in for a prolonged and daunting period of quarantine detention. Their ire turned to dismay. For Mayor Lewis, caught between the proverbial rock and a hard place, there was only one faint hope.

• • •

UNDER THE ACT OF UNION, when British Columbia joined Canada in 1871, quarantine matters suddenly became the Canadian government's responsibility. But a year later when the *Prince Alfred* hove into view with ailing Bertha Whitney on board, a federal quarantine officer had still not been appointed to the port. With no Dominion medical official, no Dominion presence was felt. Naturally, given the new federal responsibility, the provincial government refused to burden itself with the construction of a quarantine facility and the huge financial outlay such a proposal entailed.

The only existing medical facilities in Victoria at the time of the *Prince Alfred*'s arrival were two small hospitals, one built by HBC employees and the other created more recently by the city council to serve the local white European population. The so-called temporary isolation huts that had housed impoverished and dying Natives during the 1862 smallpox epidemic had been dismantled.

In 1869, after the last smallpox outbreak and just prior to the Act of Union, Dr. Trimble—then mayor of Victoria and a humanitarian—created a Board of Health, which allowed Victoria to proclaim itself a Health District and appoint a city health officer. In 1872, Mayor Lewis and his council had become ex officio members of that board. This was significant for Mayor Lewis and other succeeding officials, who now found themselves liable for all health expenses—which included underwriting the costs of all those held under quarantine thanks to Ottawa's inaction.

In spite of this, Mayor Lewis understood that the immediate need for quarantine facilities was essential. Inaction, he knew, would incur the growing wrath of common opinion that could sweep him from office. Yet action would make Victoria responsible for establishing and managing urgently needed facilities, forcing the City to take on massive new debt alone.

The one saving grace was that Victoria owned three large plots of land, which, with some effort, might serve as temporary quarantine quarters for those who were about to be detained. One was a sizable piece of open land, and the other two each contained small, wooden structures. None of these sites had ever been put to the daunting task that lay ahead.

Macaulay Point had been an HBC farm and was located in Esquimalt, west of the entrance to Victoria's Inner Harbour. Situated on a small peninsula between Harrison and Gillingham Islands, it had never been subdivided or sold after the HBC transferred its land to the Crown in 1858. The mayor suspected its flat, open aspect might provide room for some tents.

Thetis Cottage was built on the shore of Esquimalt Harbour near Dyke Point by land agent James Cooper in the 1860s. It was a part of his extensive property that reached from Victoria Harbour to the Gorge Waterway. The City acquired the acreage and its small, well-constructed log cabin after its tenants moved out in the mid-1860s.

The third site, soon to be known as the "pest house," constituted the ruins of a long-abandoned farm located on Dallas Road at Holland Point. In 1863, Dr. Trimble and George Nias requested permission to pre-empt the Point. "They believed the land was not included in the acreage signed over to Britain by the HBC and to 'stake' their claim, both men constructed buildings."[18] Dr. Trimble's stake was a tiny, unused "shanty," and he soon gave up his claim, but George Nias built a cottage, cowshed, and stable and moved in. However, D.W. Higgins, Speaker of the Legislature and eminent Victoria newspaperman, reported that the Nias farm was not on Crown land, but on Aboriginal land, which was still under negotiation. After a long legal fight over possession, Nias, too, abandoned his claim and moved to Australia in a huff. His farm soon fell into ruin. For a city council facing both wrath and near bankruptcy, this falling-down structure on Dallas Road could readily serve as the primary isolation location of those most acutely ill with infectious disease. Unfortunately, those doomed to Nias's dilapidated house were also the ones with the lowest social status and the least amount of money.

• • •

On Saturday evening, Bertha Whitney and her parents were escorted from the ship. As she was being carried to the longboat, her soiled blankets and bedding, which had covered her as she lay delirious in her cabin, were rolled into a bundle, fixed with heavy irons and thrown overboard. One alarmed first-class passenger even noted that he had seen a small mattress floating toward the shore. The *Colonist* reported that the bundle sank immediately to the bottom, "never rising to disturb the sensibilities of the public."[19] How wrong and how explosive that statement would turn out to be!

The press, quick to report any sensation connected with an outbreak of smallpox among white passengers on board the *Prince Alfred*, had a field day. Every day new dispatches appeared, each more chilling than the one before, and they put the public on the edge of panic. On Saturday, June 15, the *British Colonist* reported that smallpox had come ashore "with the little sufferer" to the George Nias house and deemed Bertha's case "the most malignant type of the terrible scourge."[20] Then, Sunday's morning paper informed an already nervous public that "the infected blankets which were thrown overboard from the *Prince Alfred* had been fished up by Indians and brought into town."[21] Their whereabouts were never revealed.

Suddenly, medical offices in Victoria were overrun by citizens demanding vaccination. As "special constables were sworn in to guard the ship and the pest house,"[22] crowds ignored queues and waiting rooms and swarmed around physicians' residences. Rumours that putrid meat had been fed to steerage passengers on the *Prince Alfred* were considered "a simple perversion of truth,"[23] but the *British Colonist* did little to dispel the story. "Everyone should be vaccinated and he should have his family vaccinated as well. Families employing Chinamen and other 'help' should see that they go through the same process lest they should bring the pestilence into the household."[24]

• • •

IN ITS SOCIAL ORGANIZATION and in the treatment of disease, Victoria simply followed the model of class separation and rank that had defined English society for hundreds of years. But during the nineteenth century, "new money" born of the industrial revolution pushed its way between old hereditary wealth and the working poor, changing a centuries-old, two-tiered social system. Ocean travel reflected these new class distinctions. First-class shipboard travel meant accommodation fit for the aristocracy. It included luxurious private cabins, the best cuisine and wines, a separate promenade deck, and personal attendants who responded to every demand. Second-class travel meant that a second son travelling to the "colonies" and perhaps a brash young entrepreneur often shared a cabin. Second class also included fine cuisine served in a separate dining room. Third class was an afterthought and strictly for the working poor. Often it was a euphemism for cabined steerage. Real steerage was little more than dormitory accommodation deep in the ship's bowels near to the steering gear. Meals could be purchased on board, but more often the passengers cooked for themselves in common pots, using foodstuffs such as bully beef and potatoes they had bought in bulk just before boarding the ship in Liverpool or Cork. It was group travel at its worst. Those forced to leave Britain this way in the mid-nineteenth century were considered little more than an embarrassment to the empire.

So it was in the treatment of disease. In a time when Britain had no universal health care, the nobility and merchant classes created their own medical facilities. New institutions such as Guy's and Middlesex Hospitals and the smallpox hospital at King's Cross reflected this self-serving mindset. In the early nineteenth century, only a few "free" hospitals were constructed for the working poor. Yet, when the sense of noblesse oblige combined itself with Christian evangelism, a few new hospitals for the indigent began to appear. St. George's Hospital in London and the Royal Infirmary of Edinburgh soon became the beacons of this humanitarian impulse.

Back in Victoria, Mayor Lewis had decided to organize the quarantine detention camps for those on the *Prince Alfred* along the same strict, historically British lines of class separation. Along with rampant racism, it was to be *the* pattern of treatment for those quarantined in British Columbia for the next eighty-five years.

Detained first-class passengers from the *Prince Alfred* would go to Thetis Cottage; those in second class and cabined third were sent to Macaulay Point. Those entirely without means and who travelled in steerage, who were already ill or very likely soon to be, such as little Bertha

Whitney and her parents, were to be delivered to the falling-down pest house on Dallas Road.

All day Saturday, June 15, the mayor and Dr. Matthews supervised the preparations of the quarantine location at Macaulay Point. It would receive the largest number of detainees. Over a dozen tents, some bought and others loaned from the city's works yard, were brought to the site. Mattresses, blankets, pillows, and other paraphernalia such as oil lamps and small tables were purchased in town, while work crews spent the day constructing a cookhouse capable of feeding over sixty people. Ropes were stretched around the compound and a force of special constables was sworn in to prevent escape and keep visitors at bay. By evening all was ready.

As twilight fell, some eighty passengers from the *Prince Alfred* were taken ashore and placed under quarantine. Sixty-five from second class were escorted to Macaulay Point, eleven of whom were women. A dozen others, who had travelled first class and had substantial social standing and influence in the city, were taken to Thetis Cottage. These included the dowager Mrs. Peter Owens, the well-known Irving sisters, and the esteemed and successful Victoria businessman Mr. McLean, his wife, and their three children. Once settled in, Mr. McLean took charge, polled his associates, and promised that he would have everything they wished for sent up to Thetis Cottage without delay. Only Bertha Whitney and her indigent parents were taken to Nias's noxious, dank, and deserted hovel on Dallas Road. With the yellow quarantine flag flying from its rooftop gable, the pest house would soon gain a fearsome reputation.

Back at Macaulay Point, members of the press jostled each other to record the arrival of its first batch of inmates. At the outset, reporters praised the mayor's efforts. "Shortly before nightfall 25 passengers were transported to Macaulay Point and took up their quarters. The poor unfortunates appeared greatly delighted, and the camp with the bonfires burning and lights flashing created a romantic scene after dark."[25] The following Monday, June 17, *British Colonist* journalists spent the whole day at Macaulay Point.

We visited the camp yesterday and found the passengers generally in excellent health and spirits. The males were smoking choice Havana cigars and occasionally "splicing the main-brace" and talking to their friends outside the ropes, who stood without.[26]

With a few good Scotches under their belts, several of the young men had moved toward a young ingénue who was seated on a trunk near one of the ladies' tents. She had a flirtatious smile, half-hidden by a huge Dolly Varden hat, and was busy cutting out prints from an illustrated paper, presumably to hang inside her tent as decoration. A long table near the cookhouse had been covered with foods of every description. Those few cabined steerage passengers who were among the Macaulay Point contingent were busy stuffing themselves, "while festive-looking Chinamen flitted to and fro supplying the wants of the other guests."[27] A young reporter smitten by the young coquette strained at the ropes to ask her how she liked the situation. "It was splendid and seemed so like a picnic on an extensive scale,"[28] she cooed.

The mayor could be seen handing out blankets and promising he would soon deliver seventy-five more, "as the nights are very cold."[29] Grinning like a Cheshire cat, Lewis had scored a major political coup. Dr. Matthews simpered about, vaccinating everyone in sight, until one adamant anti-vaccinationist refused the treatment, declaring loudly that he would knock the good doctor senseless if he tried. Although he did not press the issue, Matthews was heard to retort, "The Law is stronger than us both."[30] It wasn't, and the gentleman remained vaccine free.

As the days wore on, many more healthy passengers suspected of being carriers of smallpox were quarantined at Macaulay Point. As they waited for symptoms to appear, they indulged in evening concerts and dances organized for their benefit. Rowboats milled about on the sea below their encampment, their oarsmen offering immediate escape to anyone who could pay the modest fee. As of June 22, life at Macaulay Point was so good that no one had seized this opportunity and the oarsmen remained glum. Of the conditions at the Nias pest house, the *British Colonist* managed only one line: "The Whitney family is at the Pest House with the little girl, whose case is now not considered hopeless."[31]

As stories emerged from the quarantine camps, the Victoria press began to modify its initial wholesale support. On June 23, the *Colonist* received a letter signed by several passengers alleging that two of the officers from the *Prince Alfred* who had also been quarantined at Macaulay Point had been taking liberties with some female detainees. It was an issue "which reflected seriously upon the conduct of the officers."[32] However, because the signees were unknown to the newspaper's editors, they refused to publish it, printing only the notice of its receipt. They left its damning contents to their readers' imagination.

More serious was Magistrate Pemberton's letter denouncing the charges made by the *Daily Standard,* which accused him of refusing to swear in more police constables to augment security at Macaulay Point. Pemberton furiously defended his actions, claiming that Victoria police had more to do than simply guard the quarantine camp where they "might catch infection and spread it amongst the people in town."[33] Pemberton then blamed Mayor Lewis for placing ailing Bertha Whitney in the pest house, which he believed was outside the jurisdiction of Victoria's Board of Health.[34] The implication that little would be done for her was clear. Pemberton's charge turned out to be prophetic for the welfare of Bertha Whitney, her family, and the future of quarantine in British Columbia.

Back on the *Prince Alfred* after the sick and those suspected of contagion had been removed and detained, Officer Peter Eddy continued his enforcement of those left on board with new-found dispatch. What he witnessed widened the acrimony between him and the proud and volatile Captain Williams. Returning from one brief foray delivering messages ashore, Officer Eddy discovered that in his absence, Captain Williams had contravened quarantine legislation by rowing over to nearby HMS *Boxer* and "enquiring [to Her Majesty's naval officers] just how long this farce would last."[35]

Irritated, Officer Eddy noticed that all the ship's dirty linen had been piled up in the tethered longboat, once assigned to fetch fresh water. Captain Williams told the longboat crew to wash all the linen ashore, but they returned with their task undone. The captain repeated his order and told them not to come back until the job was finished. They cowered. Discovering this, Officer Eddy went ballistic and accused Captain Williams of inciting anarchy. He wrote, "It was nothing short of a willful act to transplant the disease from the ship to the shore, and only then would he realize his wishes that every son-of-a-bitch on shore might have smallpox."[36]

Resolute, Williams declared *he* would take the linen ashore himself. Only when Eddy threatened "that it was more than he and his ship was worth to dare"[37] did the captain back off. What the longboat crew had failed to mention was that as they came ashore, they were driven off by armed settlers who threatened violence and prosecution.

Once the sick and suspected carriers of smallpox were disembarked, the *Prince Alfred* was cleared and allowed to proceed to Nanaimo for coal. Beyond the skeleton crew, there remained a small group of Chinese steerage passengers on board who were thought to have had no contact with Bertha Whitney. Dr. Matthews's initial medical examinations proved deficient, because by the time the ship reached Nanaimo, two more cases of smallpox had broken out. The ship's second mate, Mr. Hunter, and second steward, Mr. Hall, had become seriously ill. Once in Nanaimo, and fearing the worst, Mr. Dunzall, the ship's purser; Wells Fargo agent Mr. Webster; and two others who had remained on the *Prince Alfred* in Victoria jumped ship. They found passage for Victoria on the Pacific Navigation Company's steamer *Emma*, which left Nanaimo later the same day. Other passengers, fearing the worst, also fled from the *Prince Alfred* and disappeared into the darkness of the rough-and-ready coal town. Fearing a mass exodus of everyone on board, Captain Williams immediately ordered his "lines away" and steamed south, off into the night.

The *Prince Alfred* reached Victoria a little ahead of the smaller *Emma* early on Sunday, June 21. Captain Williams rounded up and dropped anchor, this time in Victoria Harbour. Once again he ran up the yellow flag of quarantine and fired two guns to signal his arrival. Dr. Matthews appeared with dispatch and received the disturbing news. When the deserters on the *Emma* pulled up to the Dickson, Campbell & Company wharf in Victoria's Inner Harbour, Matthews had the ship met by medical officials *and* a large contingent of police. Those from the *Emma* were detained, and both it and the *Prince Alfred* were immediately placed under quarantine from four o'clock Sunday, June 23, for twenty-one days. Williams and Captain Rudlin of the *Emma* reluctantly complied, taking their vessels farther up the harbour and dropping their hooks. Rudlin, feisty like Williams, would soon fight again.

Word soon spread that other passengers who had disappeared from the *Prince Alfred* while in Nanaimo had found passage back to Victoria on board the steamer *Maude*, which was due in town that day at noon. When it arrived at the quay, the Victoria constabulary searched the vessel and found Mr. McGregor of the California Cricketers, Mr. and Mrs. Smith of the California Elevens, and several others, and took them into custody. Dunzall, Webster, and several others from the *Emma* and the *Maude* were escorted to Macaulay Point. Second Steward Hall and two others from the *Prince Alfred* were taken to the pest house.

There, in a darkened room, they saw the ailing Bertha Whitney. Fearing for his own life, Mr. Hall made a run for it. With few provisions, no treatment, and no nursing care, Bertha Whitney and her ailing parents had simply been left to die. Hall was panic-stricken. By the time he was captured, he had developed the telltale papules. When cornered, he went hysterical. With the press hot on the trail, the full horror of the pest house was about to become widely known. The *Colonist* reported, "He was half-naked, with a horribly swollen face and head, and his body was covered with a number of sores."[38] When Hall was spotted by the backyard fence of a resident of Medana Grove, residents from James Bay to Beacon Hill became so terrified of other pest house escapees that security officers guarding the place were threatened with hefty fines and imprisonment if they were charged with dereliction of duty. Luckily Hall recovered, the infection did not spread, and the threats were dropped.

Ten days had now passed since the *Prince Alfred* first arrived in Victoria. The sixty-five passengers first quarantined at Macaulay Point were by then considered past the dangerous smallpox-incubation period. When none of the detainees contracted the disease in the next four days, Dr. Matthews declared them smallpox free, and they were discharged. The most recent admissions to Macaulay Point and the pest house also remained disease free for twenty-one days, and they too were finally released.

Predictably, there was a tragic ending to this story. Though the parents of the stricken child survived the disease, their beloved little daughter died.

Bertha Whitney was buried in the grove between the pest house and the sea. Dean Cridge of Christ Church Cathedral performed the funeral.

At Holland Point on Dallas Road, a granite memorial to the sad fate of the child still stands, hidden in a copse of trees. It reads:

> *In memory of Bertha E. Whitney, aged five years, passenger on the steamship Prince Alfred, inbound from San Francisco, who died of smallpox, June 23, 1872. Other unknown victims were also buried here. The Pest House stood nearby on Dallas Road.*

The full force of Victoria's inadequate quarantine facilities had been brought home by the death of this innocent little girl. In a blistering editorial on Tuesday, June 25, 1872, the *Colonist* rightly blamed all levels of government, but demanded that concerted action be directed toward Ottawa:

> Turning to the Act of Union we find amongst the encumbered list of subjects for Federal legislation "Quarantine and the establishment and maintenance of Marine Hospitals" . . . No movement, so far as we are aware, has yet been made toward providing for the possible wants of the Province in this respect. Perhaps the appearance of smallpox may have enabled the public to realize the importance of this question.[39]

The editorial bashed both civic and provincial governments for inaction and outright ineptitude. "The prompt removal to proper quarters of the plague-stricken child and the proper and rigid treatment of the ship, passengers and crew might have prevented the spread of the disease . . . The passengers were quarantined, that is after a fashion, and a show was made of disinfecting the ship. But the whole thing was so loosely and inefficiently done that it only excited ridicule."[40]

Recounting the events at Macaulay Point, Nanaimo, and the pest house—which had become known as a "house of death"—the editorial concluded that "such a concatenation of blunders of omission and commission is difficult to explain . . . No time should now be lost in making such provisions as will enable proper and effective quarantine to be performed both here and at Nanaimo, New Westminster and Burrard Inlet . . . It is with the hope of arousing the authorities both here and at Ottawa to due diligence and a fitting sense of responsibility that the subject has been again brought before the public."[41]

• • •

WHAT MADE OTTAWA SIT up to its responsibilities in the events surrounding Bertha Whitney's death was when Mayor Lewis presented Ottawa with invoices for the costs of the *Prince Alfred* smallpox debacle. In 1868, before federal involvement, the provincial government had paid $754.50 for six claims (medical supplies, special equipment, a nurse's salary, the medical examiner's salary, post-mortems, and burial costs), to curb an epidemic that killed fifty Natives in Victoria. However, when the bills came in for the care of the *Prince Alfred* passengers, the Victoria Board of Health was aghast. Total claims against the City amounted to a whopping $12,132.67.[42]

The Dominion was not amused when Lewis calmly passed on to Ottawa a total of fifty-six claims for payment. Not only did the Victoria Board of Health submit expenses for its own treatment and services at the three quarantine camps, but they also endorsed claims submitted by certain important individual Victoria citizens who were on board the stricken ship. Some of the claims, some sixteen times greater than those of the 1868 epidemic, were so excessive that the Canadian government cried foul and ordered a commission to sort out the mess.

The Honourable Mr. Justice Gray presided. Ottawa argued that "in making themselves the self-constituted agents of the Dominion government, the [Victoria] Board of Health was bound to exercise a reasonable discretion in the incurring of expenditure sufficient to meet the exigency."[43] Ottawa asserted that Victoria had been most indiscreet and had spent lavishly, turned a blind eye to excessive spending by certain passengers, and collaborated with them in squeezing money from the Canadian government. It was easy to see why.

One of the claims that Victoria submitted was for $2,325 in wages and room and board for five special constables at Macaulay Point. Investigation soon proved that the constables were still receiving wages twelve days *after* the last of the *Prince Alfred*'s passengers had been discharged. Justice Gray adjusted the claim. Peter Eddy, the special constable on board the *Prince Alfred*, had his outrageous claim of $7.50 per day cut in half. Another claim by the Victoria Board of Health was for $337 for carriage hire to be placed at the disposal of visitors, city councillors, officers, gentlemen, and others at Macaulay Point. It too was adjusted. Justice Gray also felt that the food allowance claim of $2.50 per day for all detained passengers and personnel at Macaulay Point was another instance of "enjoyed luxuries" and far in excess of the fifty-cent daily food allowance provided to the eight Chinese passengers who were detained on board the stricken ship.

Ottawa also queried Victoria's claim for $11,114.42 for mattresses and furniture used at Macaulay Point, especially when passengers at that facility were far fewer in number than the number of beds and other items bought. Andrew Astrico, proprietor of the Pacific Telegraph Hotel in Victoria, submitted what was perhaps the most outrageous claim. The Pacific Telegraph was advertised as "the most commodious and cleanest hotel in Victoria, with meals at all hours of the day,"[44] and Mayor Lewis had hired Astrico to provide meals for all those detained at the Macaulay Point encampment. He had been initially guided by the hotel's posted charges of 37.5 cents per meal. Lewis had accepted that there would be extra charges for delivery and other incidentals. Sensing an opportunity to make some real money, Astrico had supplied all the "cabined" passengers from the *Prince Alfred*— the Chinese passengers, special constables, labourers, and servants—"with a profusion that must have astonished them."[45] The daily menu was secretly forwarded to the *Colonist* by Mr. Samuel Harris, a whistle-blowing special security constable, who claimed to be the "caterer."

— *Bill of Fare* —

DINNER QUARANTINE. SUNDAY, JUNE 30, 1872.

Chicken soup, Fish, Roast Turkey, Roast Beef,
Roast Mutton, Roast Lamb and capers
Corned Beef, Roast Tongue, Green Peas and Cabbage,
Mashed and Baked Potatoes,
Sago Pudding, Pies, raspberries, Cherries, Ice-Cream,
Ale, Porter, Claret, Punch.

—

Supplied from—The Telegraph Hotel—S. Harris, Caterer.[46]

Astrico argued that "the Mayor directed him to supply the constables with five or six drinks each day; that the ladies wanted the best wine; that claret and other wines were sent down about 5 dozen and 2 or 3 casks of beer, on the first day."[47] This continued for thirty-eight days. Beyond this, Astrico charged exorbitantly for hired men, cartage of water and provisions, personal carriage hire, wear and tear, and a $20 per diem fee for his services. It all amounted to a whopping fee of $7,390.37.

In essence, that fee meant each person at the Macaulay Point encampment was charged $9.50 per day. By comparison, the Fifth Avenue Hotel in New York City charged $5.00 per day, and the Occidental in San Francisco charged $3.50. Rates for the Driard and Colonial Hotels in Victoria were posted at $2.50.[48] For those at Macaulay Point, quarantine detention was analogous to staying at some of the best hotels in North America, despite the tents. For Astrico, quarantine had become, with the mayor's blessing, a cash cow. Justice Gray soon flushed out the rodent and awarded him a total of $1,782, one-third of his original claim.[49]

At Thetis Cottage, the first-class detention house, the situation was equally grand and equally appalling. Mr. McLean was a former American magistrate and now eminent Victoria businessman and considered "of undoubted character." He had initially refused accommodation at Macaulay Point and had demanded to be placed with several others of his social standing at Thetis Cottage. McLean submitted claims to bring the place up to the standards befitting the status of its temporary residents. Naturally, Mayor Lewis granted his request, and so he, his wife, three children, and seven others were moved to Thetis Cottage, where they remained for nine days. Invoices submitted in open court showed "every comfort and luxury of the season including fruits and wines in addition to the best of solid food was provided in abundance."[50]

In his defence, McLean told Mr. Justice Gray that he had been requested by several other American gentlemen and "guests" to spare no expense. "Thetis Cottage was put in order; a new cooking stove and utensils was bought. A cook was hired from Victoria, and everything else done that was required."[51] His claim, though adjusted, was largely allowed.

And so it went. Wholly inadequate facilities, mismanagement, poor enforcement of quarantine regulations, federal indifference, the social expectations and entitlements of class, and outright knavery were revealed before all. The three hastily arranged quarantine camps in Victoria in 1872 were shown to be completely untenable. Justice Gray had confirmed the lesson already apparent in Bertha Whitney's death—that there was no longer any excuse for the delay in the construction of a federally funded quarantine station.

Another ten years would pass before much happened. During the late 1870s, the Dominion was beside itself trying to finance the Canadian Pacific Railway (CPR), while ships inbound to Victoria full of Chinese labourers hired to construct its western route through the mountains continued to dump any human cargo showing signs of illness along the western shores of the Juan de Fuca Strait. It was a strategy used to avoid the delays and costs of sporadic quarantine inspections in Victoria. China Beach is aptly named.

Finally, in the fall of 1882, the Canadian government allocated $5,000 for the purchase of land and for the construction of a permanent, comprehensive, federally operated quarantine structure on Canada's west coast.

On August 1, 1883, eleven years after the death of Bertha Whitney, Dr. William Jackson was appointed the first dominion quarantine officer on Canada's west coast. Ottawa wanted the site to be in Esquimalt, near the naval station, and Jackson became the pitchman. Underscoring the benefit of such a presence, the federal government raised its ante to $7,500.

It did no good. For many citizens of Victoria, Esquimalt was far too close to their own gem of a city for *any* quarantine station, however lavishly funded.

Memories of the Dallas Road pest house soon fuelled a massive citizens' protest. At the time, Esquimalt was still largely unsettled, but it was designated as a proposed "suburb" and Victorians knew that they had a great deal to lose if a quarantine station sprang up in its midst. The *Colonist* backed the people:

The apparently obstinate determination of the Dominion Government, against all reason and in the teeth of the strongest representations on our part of our city members and others to locate the hospital in

Esquimalt, promises to be a very serious matter indeed to the people of this place. A pest house at the Esquimalt terminus of the Island Railway, in the very heart of what is, in a short time, destined to become an important town, is really something that cannot be justified.[52]

It did not take long for coal baron Robert Dunsmuir to come on side. The last thing he needed was a quarantine facility near his coal terminus. As a newly elected member of the provincial legislature, Dunsmuir found ready support. Dunsmuir's "energetic protests" soon joined forces with Victoria's infamous hard-line conservative mayor Noah Shakespeare. Shakespeare had witnessed the arrival of thousands of Chinese into Victoria and parlayed a growing anti-Chinese sentiment to win a seat as a federal MP. In 1883, he tabled a motion in Ottawa to prohibit Chinese immigration altogether. Dunsmuir and Shakespeare's partnership was born in hell, and it proved to be an omen of darker things to come.

Their anti-Esquimalt lobby worked. On July 10, 1884, the federal minister of public works, Hector-Louis Langevin, sent a telegram to Noah Shakespeare and others in Victoria to announce that the Albert Head Peninsula, at the northern extremity of Parry Bay, a dozen miles farther west of Victoria and well beyond the town limits of Esquimalt, would be the location of the new Dominion quarantine station.[53]

On September 19, 1884, the *Colonist* reported, "the site selected is commanding and healthy, possessing good natural drainage and has been approved by the Dominion Government agent J. W. Trutch."[54] Local contractor Charles Hayward was hired, and the building begun.

The main structure of the new Albert Head Quarantine Station was copied largely from plans used at Grosse Île. "It was a building consisting of two wings, forty-five by seventy feet, each connected by long corridors with an apartment and offices for the resident surgeon in the middle. The wings were for the patients and were to be fitted with baths, water closets, and all [the] modern necessities. It was to be constructed at the end of the long Albert Head Peninsula and would be about two hundred feet long."[55]

By January 1885, the main building was finished. Although it was $619.98 over budget, the station still required staff houses, a laboratory, disinfection buildings, a fumigation plant, a through-road to Metchosin, and an all-important wharf long enough to handle ocean-going ships. Ottawa promised that the facility would be fully equipped within the year. The one item completely ignored was the wharf. Its absence was critical, and it would dog the Albert Head Station to its end.

Nonetheless, in June 1886, with final expenditures amounting to $12,127.61, Dr. William Jackson became the first chief medical officer of the first federal quarantine station at Albert Head.

It was done. Fourteen years after the death of Bertha Whitney, British Columbia had finally acquired its own federally funded quarantine facility. At first glance, at least for Victoria's white community, it seemed that the problem of curbing incoming infectious diseases had finally been solved. Curiously, the day before the Whitneys arrived on the *Prince Alfred* in 1872, another notice appeared in the *Colonist* that should have gotten equal attention but did not:

> A CHINESE LEPER—A Chinaman afflicted with the leprosy, is lying in a dying state in the bushes just beyond Mr. Finlayson's. He presents a horrid appearance, fingers and toes dropping off at the joints, teeth falling from their sockets and with other unmistakable signs of the dread disease. His countrymen have turned him out to die, and he lies alone in his misery without the slightest covering.[56]

By the time quarantine officials finally got around to dealing with the more serious issue of leprosy among the Chinese population, it was 1891, nineteen years after the notice in the paper. Even then, it was done in a manner that would make Bertha Whitney's wretched pest house seem like a vacation resort.

CHAPTER 3 // SMALLPOX WARS: A DISASTROUS START

After we crossed the long illness that was the ocean, we sailed upstream.
On the first island the immigrants threw off their clothes
and danced like sand-flies.

—Margaret Atwood, "Further Arrivals"[1]

D r. MacNaughton-Jones should have known that the Albert Head Quarantine Station was doomed right from the start. For one thing, his predecessor, Dr. William Jackson, had not lived on-site for three years; he lived in Victoria, some eighteen kilometres away. Even Dr. Jackson knew this was the Dominion's first quarantine station on the west coast and it needed a full-time resident director—not only to enforce quarantine regulations but also to advocate for the continued improvement in infectious disease control. Those quarantined needed him on-site; the citizens of British Columbia wanted him on-site, and Ottawa ought to have paid attention. Without a chief medical officer at the helm, the new Albert Head Quarantine Station would be rudderless.

When Dr. MacNaughton-Jones succeeded William Jackson on May 31, 1890, Albert Head *still* had no resident medical director, no deep-water wharf, and no inshore quarantine steamer enabling officers to meet incoming ships at sea. The anchorage was not trustworthy in winter, and the station lacked an all-weather road to the outside world. There was no large-scale sulphur-dioxide apparatus to fumigate infected ships, no disinfecting apparatus for travellers' baggage, no proper disinfecting showers, no bacteriological laboratory, and no reliable freshwater supply. The detention hospital was still unfinished; its two-storey frame structure, designed for eighty patients, had only eight cots and "no sufficient bedding to afford a change for each."[2] The facility was understaffed, unheated, and without a fire-extinguishing system. What it had was a dozen cups and saucers in the cafeteria, but only "six knives and forks, six teaspoons, and six dessert spoons."[3] The one thing Albert Head had going for it after four years was the hospital's yellow paint, which indicated its purpose was for quarantine. Remote and almost hidden in a wilderness miles from Victoria, there was no signage, no notice that the place had anything to do with the large-scale containment of contagious diseases. These structural and operational deficiencies reached out from the Albert Head Quarantine Station like the tentacles of some giant Pacific octopus, and it turned what was a masquerade of effort into a theatre of misadventure.

When he was hired in 1890, Dr. MacNaughton-Jones had no direct experience in quarantine medicine. He did, however, come with a wealth of experience in public health and medical administration. He was born in Cork, Ireland, in 1832, and followed his brother Henry into medicine at Queen's University. After graduation and further training at St. George's Hospital in London, he immigrated to New Westminster, BC, in 1862 with his wife and young daughter, Florence. Within a year, he was elected as the representative for the district of Lillooet in the colony's Legislative Council. He was just thirty-one.

Dr. MacNaughton-Jones quickly established himself as a first-class surgeon; indeed, many of his colleagues considered him "the best in the colony."[4] In 1864, he was appointed coroner for the district of New Westminster, and in 1866, he became coroner for all of British Columbia. During this time, thousands of immigrants flooded to Vancouver Island to work in Robert Dunsmuir's Wellington Colliery in Nanaimo. Dr. MacNaughton-Jones joined the burgeoning enterprise as colliery surgeon.

In Nanaimo, he had three more children, William, George, and Helen. He and Reverend James Raynard, rector of St Paul's Anglican church, founded the Nanaimo Junior Brass Band, while his wife raised money for the uniforms of the newly formed Boys' Brigade.

In November 1874, Dr. MacNaughton-Jones moved to Victoria, "intending to take up permanent residence in that city,"[5] but instead he was appointed medical attendant in charge of the Royal Cariboo Hospital in Barkerville. He stayed there for two years before becoming the superintendent of the new provincial lunatic asylum in New Westminster in 1877. He resigned in frustration less than a year later after discovering a litany of organizational and construction faults that made the new asylum, at least for him, completely unworkable. He wrote "On the whole, the building, in its present state, seems to me a madhouse of former times, and not a modern hospital for patients affected with diseases of the brain."[6] It is surprising that his critical eye did not extend to the insanity that would soon reach pandemic proportions at Albert Head.

British Columbia was booming with its own special frenzy. Confederation had brought a rush of settlers who wished to make the province more than a just a flash in a gold pan. The completion of the CPR's west coast terminus in 1885 brought thousands from Europe, the British Isles, and eastern Canada. Many would settle on Vancouver Island, and that motivated the Canadian Pacific Navigation Company to establish a lucrative passenger, mail, and freight service across the Strait of Georgia between the mainland and Victoria. In the United States, the completion of the Great Northern Railway's spur line to Tacoma, Washington, in 1887 enabled the whole Pacific Northwest to flourish. Regular steamer service from San Francisco and Portland brought hundreds to British Columbia, while the steamships *Abyssinia*, *Batavia*, and *Parthia*, chartered by the CPR Steamship Lines in 1887, launched a prosperous trans-Pacific service.

Quarantine stations had been established in Seattle and Port Townsend in the 1880s, clearing those entering the northern states from the Pacific. But with the opening of the Albert Head Station on the Canadian side of the Juan de Fuca Strait, there was some initial jurisdictional confusion. Did ships already cleared in American ports need to be cleared again in Canadian waters?

In October 1885, the American steamer *Olympian* from Puget Sound anchored off the Albert Head Quarantine Station with a suspected case of smallpox on board. Two days later, with no one around to enforce its detention, Captain T.J. Wilson simply left. When the suspected case turned real, Wilson returned. This time his ship was detained, and Captain Wilson was brought before Victoria's police magistrate for ignoring quarantine. Rather than point to the deficit of officials at Albert Head, Wilson simply pleaded ignorance of the progression of the disease. The case was dismissed.[7] It was not an auspicious start.

The detention buildings at Albert Head remained unfurnished and the station still lacked an inspection vessel all through 1886. With outbreaks of smallpox steadily moving north from San Francisco, Albert Head remained wholly ill-equipped to prevent an epidemic from reaching Victoria. Dr. Jackson did alert his federal Department of Agriculture mandarins in Ottawa to the possible dangers, but they did nothing. In 1887, the steamer *George W. Elder* arrived in Victoria from California with a single case of measles on board. The afflicted child was removed to the station hospital, where she quickly recovered, and the ship was released.

All the while, packet steamers had been transporting undetected smallpox carriers past the American coastal quarantine stations into Puget Sound, and serious outbreaks there became more common. On January 22, 1888, the steamer *Umatilla* arrived in Victoria from San Francisco. Dr. Jackson detected a case of smallpox on board. Luckily, this case was a mild one and the patient was soon discharged; however, British Columbia's luck was fast running out.

In June 1888, the Canadian Pacific Steamship *Parthia* arrived in Vancouver from Yokohama with a second-class passenger ill with smallpox. The case had been undetected by quarantine officers at the Albert Head Quarantine Station, and in Vancouver, eight other shipboard cases developed from this single source. Medical officials contained the disease and wrote that "the smallpox [here] was pretty thoroughly stamped out;"[8] however, Vancouver City Council was becoming increasingly nervous about Albert Head.

Everything changed with the appearance of the Canadian-Pacific Navigation Company's coastal steamship *Premier* in Vancouver in January 1889. Its arrival resulted in a histrionic chain of events that came to be known as the "smallpox wars." Waged between the two long-standing rival cities of Victoria and Vancouver, the campaign lasted three years and became the means by which west coast quarantine legislation would be tested in open court and the facilities at Albert Head found wholly wanting.

On January 5, 1889, the *Premier* steamed up from Seattle to Vancouver by way of Admiralty Inlet, Rosario, and Georgia Strait. Already cleared at the Seattle Quarantine Station, Captain O'Brien did not divert to Albert Head some twelve kilometres east on the Juan de Fuca Strait, but proceeded directly to the mainland city. Upon reaching Vancouver, the city's chief medical officer, Dr. Beckingsale, received the *Premier's* American clearance papers and went aboard. There he spotted an active case of smallpox and ordered the ship to proceed immediately to the Albert Head Quarantine Station. Sensing that the *Premier* may not comply with his order, the doctor remained on board while Captain O'Brien reluctantly left Vancouver and pointed his ship down the Strait of Georgia toward the faraway station beyond Victoria in Parry Bay.

At Albert Head, there being no wharf, the *Premier* dropped anchor and waited. With no inshore station launch or medical officers to pick him up, Dr. Beckingsale now found himself trapped on board a quarantined vessel. He was furious. Others who had had no contact with the smallpox sufferer denounced the steamship company over the trains they had failed to catch in Vancouver. For seven days, the *Premier* rolled uneasily on the exposed seas. Dr. Beckingsale vaccinated passengers as needed, but he was unable to establish regular communication with medical officials at the station. Time passed slowly. Then, on January 12, a frustrated Captain O'Brien ordered his crew to weigh anchor and steam away toward Vancouver. This act broke federal law.

When news reached Vancouver that the *Premier* had left Albert Head without proper quarantine clearance, Mayor David Oppenheimer, nervous about contagion spreading to Vancouver from Puget Sound, believed that a Vancouver bylaw could prohibit the ship from landing. Anticipating trouble, he placed a force of police constables at the steamer's wharf in Burrard Inlet.

The Canadian Pacific Navigation Company officers claimed Vancouver had no jurisdiction to prohibit the *Premier's* movements and interfere with its paying passengers, and they threatened an injunction against the City. In the meantime, as the ship gently slid toward the wharf, Captain O'Brien suddenly turned it away and tied up against the CPR ship *Parthia,* anchored nearby. Oppenheimer's armed contingent of police, augmented now with angry citizens, refused to allow Dr. Beckingsale and others to leave the ship. They ordered it untied at once. O'Brien hesitated, then yielded. In the middle of the melee, he had secured permission to go over to Moodyville on the north shore and take on water. There, two passengers, including Dr. Beckingsale, jumped ship. At that point, they too broke federal law.

The night of January 12, the Canadian Pacific Navigation Company ship *Islander,* under the command of the affable Captain George Rudlin, sailed over from Victoria along with company president John Irving. Once in Burrard Inlet, Captain Rudlin came alongside the anchored *Premier,* and under the direction of his superior, transferred most of its passengers to his own ship. With passengers from both ships now completely intermingled on the *Islander,* Vancouver health officials had their work cut out for them in separating one from the other. Confident in the deviousness of this move, Irving then ordered Rudlin to head his ship directly for the nearby CPR quay.

The ploy, however, had been spotted by Oppenheimer's special constables. Suddenly, Rudlin, under instructions from Irving, wheeled the *Islander* to the Hastings Mill Wharf (site of the old Centennial Pier), only to do an about-face and head back to the CPR quay. Vancouver police, along with their reinforcements, began their "Keystone Cops" chase from wharf to wharf, determined to resist the *Islander*'s attempts to land at every turn.

Captain Rudlin changed course again and headed his ship directly for the shore. As described in *The Princess Story,* by Norman Hacking and W. Kaye Lamb, "At the CPR Wharf, a gangway was unexpectedly run out from the ship, and led by company president Irving and Captain Rudlin, a number of passengers rushed for the dock."[9] A scuffle ensued, and the police commissioner ordered the Vancouver Fire Department to turn its hoses on the crowd. Outraged, Irving screamed for the *Islander*'s own hoses to be fired upon the firefighters. Before it ended, several Vancouver citizens and *Islander* passengers were injured. "Loud and fierce protests and denunciations were hurled from the deck of the vessel,"[10] proclaimed the *Vancouver News-Advertiser*, but profanities alone were not enough to save the day.

Captain Irving demanded Mayor Oppenheimer return to Victoria to settle the issue. The mayor ignored him. Threats of lawsuits between the two cities ensued, and the Victoria-based Canadian Pacific Navigation Company ultimately filed an injunction against Vancouver's edict. The suit and its demand for $50,000 in damages eventually withered and was finally withdrawn. Dr. Beckingsale, however, had some very serious explaining to do.

What made this melodrama particularly alarming was that the underlying deadly reality of smallpox had once again reached British Columbia. Moreover, the lack of facilities and procedures at the Albert Head Quarantine Station suddenly came into sharp focus. Without a proper deepwater wharf capable of landing passengers, an inshore tender, or adequate fumigating equipment, it seemed vessels ordered into quarantine could simply do as they pleased.

Dominion quarantine legislation and its enforcers on the west coast had proven powerless to intercede when the rules were broken. Worse, local bylaws were simply not strong enough to chasten maritime entrepreneurs who put profit before passenger safety and public health. Although the gnashing of teeth between the two cities eventually quieted, the whole *Premier* incident became a portent of more serious tensions between Victoria and Vancouver over issues of quarantine inspection and control.

This first skirmish in the smallpox wars was to become a moment of truth for the Albert Head Quarantine Station. Bureaucrats in Ottawa could bring the facility up to the same standards as eastern stations, or they could continue to proffer empty promises. They chose the latter. In the meantime, larger and larger ocean ships, some full of deadly contagion, continued to steam for our shores.

Dr. Jackson resigned his position at the Albert Head Quarantine Station on May 31, 1890. His three years had accomplished little. The next day, Dominion quarantine officer Dr. MacNaughton-Jones became its chief medical administrator and he began an immediate campaign to rid British Columbia of ship-borne infectious diseases and restore the tarnished reputation of Albert Head. If he was not able to live on-site, he would at least attack the station's deficiencies directly from Victoria—and that attack, he hoped, would come through his own rigorous interpretation and application of Canadian quarantine law.

By the early 1890s, American inshore steamers bound for Victoria or Vancouver largely ignored the Albert Head Quarantine Station. Instead, they carried clearance from quarantine facilities on the American side of the Juan de Fuca Strait. This was not good enough for MacNaughton-Jones, so he began boarding those American vessels as they landed in Victoria to disembark passengers. "Daily steamers arriving from Puget Sound and the adjacent islands have, hitherto, been regarded as coastwise and are not reported," he wrote. "I have, however, boarded them as often as practicable, and have furnished their captains and pursers with health certificates, which they present at the customs and land passengers at their peril."[11] He added, "I have given directions that in case of any illness or death I must be notified before passengers are allowed to land."[12] Frustrated with the cavalier, though legal, attitude of American steamers that continued to slip into smaller British Columbia ports without Canadian quarantine clearance, MacNaughton-Jones added, "I can only render of what I am cognizant."[13]

Dr. MacNaughton-Jones also urged federal regulators to adopt the American quarantine regulation requiring compulsory vaccination for all Chinese passengers bound from Asia to cities on America's west coast. He argued, "I think if this rule was generally known and inflexibly adopted the public would soon acquiesce. Now would be the time to promulgate the rule; later on the change might not be easy or feasible."[14] Knowing that MacNaughton-Jones was new to his position, Ottawa coolly ignored his demands.

During MacNaughton-Jones's first six months on the job, he had his officers examine 917 vessels. Of these, ninety-eight were coastal steamers docked at Albert Head's temporary outer wharf in Victoria, and the rest, including ten sailing ships, were from across the Pacific. In total, he cleared 19,716 passengers and crew.[15] Working from Victoria, he wrote to Ottawa that he paid "visits of surprise to Albert Head, 14 miles distant, at least once a month and . . . always found the hospital clean." It was clean because it was underused. He ended his first annual report with a codicil stating that the interior of the hospital building still required repairs.

MacNaughton-Jones could not sustain the pace of his inspections while stationed in Victoria and, at the same time, oversee the steady increase in quarantine detentions at Albert Head. Despite his efforts, procedures at the station had deteriorated within two years to the point where mainland citizens were becoming alarmed. Soon, people were demanding the station be closed.

In late December 1891, the CPR steamship *Empress of China* arrived at the Albert Head Quarantine Station's wharf in Victoria Harbour. Only one passenger, a Mrs. Livingstone, travelling second class, drew medical attention. She was reported as having only a case of "hysteria," so the ship was duly cleared and allowed to proceed to Vancouver. Four days later, Mrs. Livingstone developed the telltale papules of smallpox. When Vancouver health officer Dr. Carroll visited her onboard the *Empress* in Vancouver, he observed that the eruptions were already three days old and stated that the case "should have been detected *before* the vessel came into port."[16]

Immediately, both she and the *Empress of China* were returned to the Albert Head Quarantine Station. Dr. Carroll's rigour had saved Mrs. Livingstone's life. Her active case of smallpox was treated and she survived, but it had turned out to be the worst type, confluent smallpox, which left her with permanent disfiguring scars. In the meantime, all the other passengers had been landed and vanished into Victoria or continued on to their respective mainland destinations.

Seven months later, in late April 1892, Joseph Reid began to feel desperately ill. He had been hired by CPR steamships to watch over a group of Chinese "coolies" who had arrived in steerage on the *Empress of Japan* at the Albert Head Quarantine Station on April 17 on their way to Vancouver. On that Pacific crossing, a case of smallpox had broken out among them, but this time it was detected. Decisively, Dr. MacNaughton-Jones had all 540 passengers removed from the ship and detained. Still half-finished, the Albert Head Quarantine Station was not equipped to handle such a number, so while many were directed to the unfurnished Chinese detention house, many more were put in tents. Angered at these arrangements,

MacNaughton-Jones wrote "they were all vaccinated and fumigated *to the best of my powers . . . [T]he ship was cleansed as far as possible with the means at my command* [author's emphasis]."[17]

The implication was clear: MacNaughton-Jones wanted Ottawa to know how impossible it was to fumigate an ocean liner on an anchorage without a portable sulphur-dioxide blast apparatus, an inshore tender, and sufficient manpower to adequately carry out the job. Somehow, the 540 Chinese "coolies" coped at Albert Head for ten days under medical surveillance and were released. Joseph Reid was hired to bring them into Victoria on a scow provided by the CPR.

Once in Victoria, many Chinese simply disappeared into the city's Chinatown. Reid, along with a friend by the name of Mr. Hyde, rounded up as many as he could and transported them to Vancouver on the Canadian Pacific Navigation Company vessel *Islander*. Soon after, Hyde moved on to work in a logging camp in Howe Sound. He fell deathly ill a short time later, and several of his workmates developed smallpox and died.

The situation became even more ominous when it was discovered that several Caucasian passengers from that April 1892 arrival of the *Empress of Japan* had not been detained at Albert Head Station and that two of them had moved on to Vancouver. Later in June, when the *Empress of Japan* returned to Victoria, a Chinese steerage passenger developed smallpox four or five days *after* many of his countrymen were released. Luckily, he was found and quarantined in Victoria, and a few others were rounded up and detained. However, the *Empress of Japan* was not able to proceed to the quarantine station as directed because the captain reported "all her machinery had been taken to pieces."[18] The ship was summarily fumigated where it stood. Its crew was simply taken off the ship for fifteen days.

On July 8, 1892, the *Empress of China*, en route to Vancouver from Yokohama, reported to the Albert Head Quarantine Station for clearance. Aware of the growing disaffection for the station, Dr. MacNaughton-Jones gave this ship a very close inspection. He found all first-class passengers in perfect health. Indeed, they were tanned, had played deck games, and had "tripped the light fantastic" across the blue Pacific on the new liner with ample vintage wines, a French menu, and a fine orchestra. One passenger on that trip was twenty-six-year-old Rudyard Kipling. He was with Carrie, his new wife. Reporters found him "only a whit more polite" than on a previous trip he had taken as a bachelor in 1889, but he refused to say where they had been or how long they had stayed. Asked what he would write about next, he replied dismissively, "Whose business is that I wonder?"[19] The 274 Chinese passengers who had voyaged with them far below in steerage were pale but declared disease free.

However, one death had occurred on the crossing. Daniel Tauder, the boatswain's mate, had died suddenly en route of an unspecified "internal" disease. Was it smallpox or, worse, cholera? It was impossible to ascertain, because the *Empress of China*'s physician had him immediately buried at sea.

That same day, July 8, both the *Gazette* and the *British Colonist* carried a rare full-page announcement of British Columbia's quarantine regulations. Victoria citizens scrutinized it with confusion:

1. Quarantined persons will be held in special hospitals and hospital tents provided for the reception and care of the sick until the period of incubation of the disease shall have lapsed.
2. There will be proper guarding of quarantine houses, with severe penalties to be imposed where officers in charge fail to do their duty.
3. Land, unoccupied buildings, etc., will be appropriated where necessary for hospitals and quarantine buildings, the same being not less than 150 from an inhabited dwelling.
4. The inspection of all baggage and merchandise travelling with suspected travellers will take place.

These regulations, along with other restrictions, were signed by BC's premier, Theodore Davie.

Rudyard Kipling had blithely sailed into a crisis. Not amused, he set about trying to get tickets on the transcontinental train from Vancouver, promising to "grumble and kick hard if unable to obtain a lower berth."[20] The Kiplings made their getaway in the nick of time.

On Tuesday, July 12, 1892, the *British Colonist* reported that the city was in the grip of yet another severe outbreak of smallpox. To calm its readers' growing anxiety, the paper stated that the health authorities "had it well in hand," although the column contained a more ominous announcement. "Medical men were invited to meet the members of the provincial cabinet at the premier's private office on July 9."[21] The next day, it was revealed that a new smallpox quarantine station would be constructed adjacent to the Royal Jubilee Hospital. Sensing the rebuff, Ottawa reported a few days later that "Albert Head will be made equal to all the requirements of a first-class quarantine station."[22]

Within days, Victoria City Council began restricting the activities of its citizens. All meetings of the Salvation Army were banned, its meeting house closed, and staff confined to their barracks. All scheduled summer picnics and other holiday gatherings were cancelled. Victoria's isolation houses such as Ross House were given extra guards who "faced severe penalties for failing to do their duty."[23] Patients wishing admission to Royal Jubilee Hospital for unrelated medical problems were to "remain outside the grounds" until examined by a medical officer. All clothing deemed to have been in contact with any smallpox sufferer was to be immediately disinfected or burned, and those caught with any such articles were themselves ordered into quarantine. Most severe of all was the edict that vaccination for all citizens was declared compulsory.[24]

Directives escalated quickly. Suddenly, High Mass at the Roman Catholic cathedral scheduled for Wednesday, July 13, was cancelled. The downtown Clarence Hotel, which housed a suspected carrier, was quarantined. Steps were taken to remove small children from the Protestant Orphans' Home, and on Thursday, July 14, the Methodist and Presbyterian missions in Victoria were closed. The same day, the people of Revelstoke, an isolated railway town near the Alberta border, offered to take Premier Davie's family until the "dangerous outbreak" had passed. On Friday, it was announced "the offices of Doctors Hannington, Hasell, Helmcken and Davie would be open for vaccination and that all persons who could pay the dollar fee were expected to do so."[25] By week's end, the fear of smallpox was once again so palpable in Victoria that banks in the city began to fumigate paper money.

Across the strait on the mainland, Vancouver citizens learned of Victoria's newest epidemic through the *News-Advertiser*. It carried the Victoria health officer's bulletin verbatim:

Three new cases were reported at my office today, one of these was an Indian who was removed from his lodgings in Stronach Cabins to Jubilee Quarantine Station. There have been four deaths so far; 2 last night . . . J. Giles of 106 Yates Street and the woman "Georgie" at the refuge Home. Both were buried before daylight this morning [July 13]. There are now 47 cases officially reported.[26]

By week's end, fifty-six active cases of smallpox had been reported. When Victoria papers noted that two Chinese people in the convalescent stage of smallpox had disappeared, Vancouver health officials checked their statistics for signs that the disease may be spreading. When they learned that four deaths and five active cases of smallpox had already occurred in Vancouver, alarm was met with indignation. Vancouver City Council, already unsure of the efficacy of the Albert Head Quarantine Station, was coerced into action when the City of Seattle suddenly issued them an ultimatum. Either Vancouver would forbid all passenger and freight traffic from Victoria or all trade between Seattle and Vancouver would cease.

Vancouver acted immediately. With the approval of City solicitor Alfred Hamersley and the support of the New Westminster and Nanaimo councils, Vancouver passed an ordinance that had the air of an imperial proclamation. The City of Vancouver quarantined the whole city of Victoria.

On July 13, Victoria's *British Colonist* carried the news:

THE PORT QUARANTINED.

Telegraphic advices were received from Vancouver yesterday, stating that from 11 o'clock in the morning a strict quarantine has been declared against Victoria, and further, that the Vancouver Board of Health was co-operating with those of Seattle, New Westminster and Nanaimo, in the endeavor to shut off traffic between these ports and this city.[27]

In one fell swoop, Vancouver shut out Victoria from mainland life. Victoria's growing profile as a tourist destination and its civic pride as British Columbia's capital city would be ruined. It was now a city under siege, surrounded and constrained by impregnable walls. Those from Victoria who tried to land on the mainland faced an immediate two-week confinement. Such action would have catastrophic implications. The outflow of island goods through Victoria to the mainland would grind to a halt as all merchandise was subject to rigorous disinfection. With similar action begun by Seattle and Port Townsend, the whole trading area of Puget Sound and the American Pacific Northwest would be thrown into chaos. Moreover, Victoria's mail service would be subjected to fumigation with its attendant twenty-four-hour delay.

This was cheerless stuff, and Victoria's citizens sputtered with resentment. "Vancouver exhibits a spirit of malevolence that surprises even Victorians,"[28] ran the headlines. Name-calling between the two cities began, with the *Colonist* leading the charge. "Had the Victoria Board of Health, a few weeks ago, declared a quarantine against *Vancouver*, it is safe to say there would be no disease here."[29] The paper reported the case of a Vancouver woman whose infected clothing was sent to Victoria to be altered rather than fumigated or destroyed. "They were fumigated," Vancouver shot back. "Perhaps they were," The *Colonist* retorted, "but fumigation of clothing is not enough."[30]

Soon recriminations were everywhere. Angry Victoria citizens charged that Vancouver officials had imported infected sugar to the island when a nurse from Vancouver was allowed to travel freely there just prior to the outbreak. Vancouver mayor Frederick Cope, remembering the *Premier* incident three years before, sensed that the Canadian Pacific Navigation Company would again ignore the quarantine order and was likely to run its regularly scheduled sailing of the *Yosemite* into Vancouver the next day, so he telegraphed a terse message to F.W. Vincent, assistant manager of the company, and forwarded his communiqué to the *News-Advertiser*. They printed the gist of it in their July 13 morning edition:

THE YOSEMITE TO ARRIVE.

Her passengers will be prevented from landing by sheer force.

Yesterday, a dispatch was sent to the Canadian Pacific Navigation Company at Victoria by the Mayor, stating that passengers would not be allowed to land off the steamer in the morning under any conditions.

Then, outdoing Mayor Cope, the *News-Advertiser* printed the company's response:

VICTORIA, JULY 12, 1892.

Steamer will leave here tonight at the usual hour after strictly complying with all quarantine regulations now in force. According to law, we have the right to land passengers, mail, and cargo. If the landing is refused, application will be made to the Court for a mandatory injunction against the City of Vancouver who will be held responsible for damages.

—F.W. VINCENT, ASSISTANT MANAGER

• The second salvo of the smallpox wars had begun. By the time the *Yosemite* arrived in Vancouver mid-morning on Wednesday, July 13, it was estimated that a crowd of one hundred armed and angry citizens were already on the wharf in Burrard Inlet. Fearing another riot, Alfred Hamersley advised Mayor Cope and his council that police intervention might be necessary for crowd control. Vancouver Justice A.N. Richards concurred, and Vancouver Police Chief McLaren, "with a strong force of assistants," was instructed to uphold the law. He stationed his men at both the CPR landing stage and the Union Steamships wharf. The Vancouver Fire Department was again called, and fifteen men and their fire wagons were instructed to be ready to move at a moment's notice.

A replay of the *Premier* incident of January 1889 had begun, only this time its consequences for the Albert Head Quarantine Station and detention legislation would be far more severe.

Captain George Rudlin, older and more stylish now "with his new side-whiskers,"[31] took charge of the *Yosemite*. This time, when the old sternwheeler and her fifty passengers came into view around Vancouver's Prospect Point, city officials were poised to pounce.

Vancouver health officers had boarded the harbour tug *Skidegate* and moved toward the *Yosemite* as it slowed. Warned not to land, Captain Rudlin quietly ignored the order and resolutely ghosted his ship to an empty mooring buoy some three hundred yards from the city's shore. In full view of the crowd, Captain Rudlin then lowered a lifeboat, and in climbed four men: the captain, *Yosemite*'s purser J.W. Moore, *Victoria News* reporter R.A. Rannock, and Victoria resident H.E. Crossdaile, who had booked passage to England on a steamer in New York and was desperate to make his connection. Rudlin took the oars and pulled the longboat toward the shore. At the slip, Moore, still seated, handed papers signed by Victoria health officer Dr. Milne to Police Chief McLaren, who passed them on to Vancouver's health officer Joseph Huntley, who examined them carefully. After a tense moment, Huntley looked up and spoke directly to the anxious captain. He stated emphatically that notwithstanding the clean bills of health, the *Yosemite*, under no conditions, would be allowed to tie up at the wharf and no one would be allowed to land.

Pressed by Rudlin, Mr. Huntley agreed to allow the obedient and vaccinated crew to unload the *Yosemite*'s freight. Back on board, Rudlin fired up his boilers, cleared the mooring, and brought his ship alongside the quay, which had already been cleared by the Vancouver police. As the freight gangway was slid out onto the wharf, Huntley distributed disinfectant to be swilled among the cargo. With police everywhere, order seemed to prevail —at least for the moment.

Suddenly things changed. *Yosemite* passenger John Spinks made a running leap from the main deck onto the wharf. He was caught by police and unceremoniously thrown back on board. Undeterred, Spinks dusted himself off, moved to the seaward side of the ship, and lowered a lifeboat with a friend. He disappeared across the Inlet into the anonymity of the city. Moments later, the police arrested Spinks's two sons and two fishermen in a passing skiff when they attempted a similar move. From the decks of the *Yosemite*, angry Victoria passengers hurled insults at the police and any other Vancouverites within earshot.

The next day, July 14, Captain Rudlin, boldly fired up his boilers and guided the *Yosemite* eastward beyond Vancouver's jurisdiction to Port Moody. There, he put all of his passengers safely ashore. Asked later where exactly he had landed his passengers, Rudlin only smiled and replied, "Omaha."[32]

In the meantime, the provincial lieutenant-governor, Hugh Nelson, issued an order-in-council, requiring all Victoria citizens travelling to the mainland to be examined, show proof of such examination, and then be certified smallpox free. The Canadian-Pacific Navigation Company, heartened by Nelson's edict, believed that this statement superseded Vancouver's municipal ordinance and immediately made plans to ferry another shipload of passengers to Vancouver.

George Rudlin readily accepted new travellers. He called Dr. Watt, Victoria's health officer, to examine each of the *Yosemite*'s passengers, vaccinate them where necessary, and give each a clean bill of health. His company also filed an injunction against the City of Vancouver through Vancouver Island's Supreme Court Justice, Henry Pering Pellew Crease. It ordered that the *Yosemite*'s Vancouver-bound passengers be landed. Once that was done, Captain Rudlin posted the time of his ship's departure.

A heavy summer downpour greeted the *Yosemite* as it slid into Burrard Inlet on Saturday, July 16. The landing stage was already filled with a drenched and resentful mob. Again, police cleared the quay. Vancouver quarantine officers reiterated their position, stating that if any passengers landed, they would be quarantined. Again, Rudlin lowered a lifeboat, and this time six passengers were rowed ashore. Ostensibly, they had accepted Vancouver's conditions. Mrs. Trapp, whose husband and two children were already detained in Vancouver from a previous quarantine order, had decided to join him. Her travelling companion, Miss Alicia Wallace, decided to enter detention with her. Four other male passengers —Norman Stoker, John Mackie, Mr. Jenns, and Major George Bowack— decided to land and face arrest. As they were being led off, it was reported "that several of these white passengers objected strongly to be housed with Orientals."[33] Major Bowack, with commanding military authority, insisted that he and Mr. Jenns be given rooms to themselves. It was not to be. They were taken to ramshackle cabins, or "pest houses," on Hastings Street and detained in quarantine.

In the meantime, John Spinks, who had disappeared by rowboat from the *Yosemite* three days earlier, had been found and arrested. But he did better than Major Bowack and was consigned to Vancouver's gleaming new pest house for fourteen days. Back at the wharf, City solicitor Hamersley had informed Captain Rudlin that if he became involved with any further attempt to land passengers, he would be arrested. Rudlin and his ship left for Victoria. Three days later, the *Islander,* with Captain Irving as senior officer, "called at Vancouver in the course of a tourist cruise to Alaska."[34] Again, no passengers were allowed ashore, though civic authorities demanded Irving present his ship's papers for quarantine clearance.

When the *Yosemite* arrived back in Vancouver later the same day with *another* load of passengers, Captain Rudlin was served with a summons. A week later, upon his return from Alaska, the feisty Irving tried to put a few *Islander* passengers ashore. He too was threatened with arrest.

Meanwhile, the Canadian Pacific Navigation Company's application for an injunction from Supreme Court Justice Crease had been granted. It overruled Vancouver's bylaw and restrained the City from interfering with the landing of passengers from company ships. Emboldened, company officials made another application to Justice Crease "to commit the civic officials of Vancouver for contempt."[35] Were it not for the presence of a deadly smallpox epidemic waging in their midst, the whole affair might have grown wearisome in its repetition.

In the meantime, Major Bowack and several other English "gentlemen" were detained and left fuming in a crowded waterfront pest house. Far beneath their perceived positions of privilege, Bowack and the others had to prove that they were not carriers of the deadly contagion by remaining free from smallpox for fourteen days. An infuriated Bowack refused to wait, and what he did next would astound British Columbians and move the smallpox wars to a whole new level.

Major George Bowack, along with Mr. Jenns, applied to the Supreme Court of British Columbia for an immediate, absolute release on the grounds of habeas corpus. Bowack evoked one of the most powerful statutes of English common law. Dating from before Magna Carta, habeas corpus was *the* fundamental right in safeguarding the freedom of the individual against arbitrary and unlawful actions of the state. It meant that in countries where English law had sway, a prisoner had the right to raise doubts about the legality of his confinement. Literally, habeas corpus means "you shall have the body." It became a shorthand legal term for the lengthier phrase, "you have the prisoner, now bring him before me so we can judge the legality of his imprisonment." If a petition for habeas corpus was successful, a judge issued a writ for the prisoner to appear and state his case. George Bowack was full of confidence.

These two cases, the Canadian Pacific Navigation Company's application for contempt against the City of Vancouver and George Bowack's writ of habeas corpus, were significant in that the strength of existing municipal and provincial regulations would now be tested in the highest courts of the province. More important, through these charges the whole federal operation of the Albert Head Quarantine Station would be brought under close public scrutiny. The resulting outcry from all quarters would end the smallpox wars and bring the makeshift, ill-equipped station to its knees.

It is uncertain whether Major George Bowack was ever a major in the British Army, or if he assumed the appellation to add legitimacy to his recent status as a member of the Age of Elegance. Either way, this so-called English aristocrat had the right and the money to prove he was not going to be pushed around, especially by upstart Canadians.

George Bowack was a successful London merchant. He had been on a business trip to Australia and had continued on west, around the world, arriving in Victoria on July 13; he was scheduled to leave from Vancouver two days later to catch the train to Montreal and thence his ship home. Bowack had missed his train and his boat. He was not a happy man.

Victoria citizens revelled in Major Bowack's mettle. His case, after all, was theirs. "Such imprisonment," they bristled, "was intolerable in a Barbarous, much less in a free country."[36] How could an ill-conceived act of a municipal government take precedence over the historically cherished right of a free British citizen? Supreme Court Justice John Foster McCreight read Bowack's petition, and his judgment was both bewildering to the citizens of Victoria and a thunderbolt to the plaintiffs.

McCreight's ruling was that he could not rule, and it was based on a technical and historical point of law. When the Colony of Vancouver Island and the Colony of British Columbia joined in 1866, the court systems of each were separate. They were not united until 1873. By 1880, British Columbia's four Supreme Court justices had divided their jurisdiction. Justices Begbie and Crease served Vancouver Island, while Robertson and McCreight presided on the mainland. Where cases overlapped, each looked to the others for pertinent details as recorded in the records, or Supreme Court "Rolls." McCreight believed, rightly, that Justice Crease's judgment in Victoria on the Canadian Pacific Navigation Company's injunction "covered the question as to the regulations governing [Bowack's] Habeas Corpus case."[37] If Justice McCreight found Justice Crease had granted the injunction, then the habeas corpus case before him was superfluous. If Crease had denied the injunction, then McCreight could hear Bowack's petition on its own merit.

The trouble was that McCreight had no record of Crease's decision because it had not been filed in the Supreme Court "Rolls." McCreight wrote, "I must repeat what the late Master of the rolls said. He could not act on a case unless a report of it was produced."[38] Communication being slow at the time, Crease's reporting had not reached the all-important "Rolls" in time. McCreight dismissed Bowack's petition, leaving him languishing and fuming with others of lesser status in a dank quarantine cell.

A group of prominent Victoria merchants were outraged, and petitioned Premier Davie to strike down Vancouver's bylaw. They were beside themselves when the premier admitted that even *he* could not override the law. Business in Victoria had stagnated, thanks to both the epidemic of smallpox in their midst and the effects of the quarantine embargo placed around it.

Two Victoria businesses *did* make a killing, though, one more strangely than the other. Chemist shops did a roaring trade selling disinfectants, while local cigar stores could not keep their products on the shelves. Many believed that the acrid smoke of the squat, torpedo-shaped cylinder of rolled tobacco was itself a germicide.

Undaunted and still seething in his fetid detention cell, Major Bowack somehow appealed, and Justice Walkem agreed to hear his case. Bowack's lawyers argued that his arrest and detention were illegal on three grounds: first, Victoria was not an *infected locality* rife with smallpox when Bowack arrived; second, the major had complied with all quarantine regulations; and third, in arresting him, the City of Vancouver actually broke the wording of its own bylaw.

Bowack's detention was necessary, Vancouver lawyers argued, because Victoria had been designated as an *infected locality*, meaning that 1 to 2 percent of the total population was infected with the disease. The most recent census showed Victoria having some fifteen thousand residents, which would have meant three hundred cases of the disease. However, as of July 13, Victoria had only fifty active cases,[39] thus Walkem ruled that the term *infected locality* was a misnomer and unnecessarily exaggerated the danger. "Take a village of 100+ inhabitants," he wrote. "Would a respected physician pronounce it to be an 'infected locality' if two or even five happened to have smallpox?"[40]

Justice Walkem believed that "Bowack seemed himself, to have dreaded the disease, and as far as possible kept out of its way."[41] He was vaccinated immediately upon his arrival and obtained a medical certificate to that effect. His two-night stay at the Driard Hotel, he believed, could not be read as direct exposure in that "the germs of the disease may be in this courtroom. But would any sensible person say that on a mere surmise, every one of us in this court room should be marched off as suspects?"[42] Bowack's attorneys smiled. Walkem continued.

The City of Vancouver bylaw stated that "The Medical Officer shall have power to stop, detain, and examine every person coming from a place infected with a pestilential or infectious disease, in order to prevent the introduction of same into the City."[43] But Walkem revealed that Bowack had been detained *without* examination. What was the point of an examination "when it is impossible to discover whether a person has the disease until it actually had broken out . . . and that takes 14 days to incubate."[44] If that were the case, Judge Walkem asserted, only *patients* with the disease could be examined. Bowack was not a patient, and therefore Vancouver had acted beyond the limitations of its own bylaw. The justice ordered Bowack's immediate release and gave him costs associated with his detention.

• In the act of detaining Major Bowack, the City of Vancouver had ignored Justice Crease's granting of the injunction. Crease bluntly stated that such defiance amounted to contempt of court, and with that his lordship issued a writ of arrest for the mayor and members of his council.

The *British Colonist* said it all: "The City officials 'wanted' by the sheriff were arrested at a late hour last night, and were confined in the Hotel Vancouver."[45] With that, the good citizens of Vancouver went berserk. On Friday, July 23, bells were rung throughout the city to call citizens to

Market Hall for a mass protest. As the crowd swelled, a brass band kept enthusiasm "at a proper pitch." On a podium, the good reverend G.H. Maxwell condemned Justice Crease's action as "infamous and insulting," and declared that Crease himself should be quarantined. "No doubt," he went on, "enough money could be collected from Crease's insects to keep him sweet for 14 days."[46]

* The editor of the *Vancouver Daily World* further enflamed the crowd by suggesting they petition the new prime minister, John Thompson. Instead, it was decided that the steamer *Comox* would take Mayor Cope, City Solicitor Hamersley, and Medical Officer Huntley to Victoria, and that "we accompany them to the boat with a brass band and give them a proper send-off."[47] Amid much triumphant confusion, the crowd then set off for the Hotel Vancouver. With music and jubilation in the air, it was not quite anarchy, but it *was* the next best thing.

In spite of all the indignation, citizens on both sides of the Gulf were deathly afraid of the smallpox that had flowered in their midst. It was Victoria's federal MP, E.G. Prior, who understood who was to be blamed. On July 13, he had fired off a pointed telegram to Prime Minister Abbott, John Thompson's predecessor.

HON. SIR JOHN ABBOTT, OTTAWA: *Quarantine matters here at a standstill (stop). No proper means of fumigating vessels yet, though two steamships already arrived with smallpox on board (stop). Please authorize purchase or lease of suitable vessel at once (stop).*
—E.G. PRIOR.[48]

Ottawa must have been reading the Victoria papers, because two days later, on July 15, 1892, Dr. MacNaughton-Jones received word that a local steamer, *Earle,* was to be examined to see if it could serve as a quarantine boat for the Albert Head Quarantine Station. Ottawa even offered a sulphur-dioxide fumigation apparatus to be placed at MacNaughton-Jones's convenience. The *Colonist* reported, "Once the boat is secured and the dioxide machine is placed in position [onboard], it will be comparatively easy to thoroughly disinfect all ships arriving in port."[49] It took six weeks for the blast machine to be mounted on the *Earle* and tested on the old barque

Dominion anchored in Victoria Harbour. Within ten minutes, the "defunct vermin" had piled up within the ship. Yet Ottawa's belated actions were not timely enough to quell the growing anger over the smallpox debacle that waged in their midst.

On Sunday, July 25, two days after Vancouver's riotous demonstration, the city's pulpits were full of self-righteous malice toward Justice Crease and his writ of arrest for Vancouver officials. Reverend Pedley knew his embittered flock well, and Crease's action fired his own distaste *and* his eloquence. From his pulpit, Pedley's oratory would rise and fall, like that of the best of the Welsh Methodists. He began:

> *I look upon it as a public calamity. When you cannot trust your pilot, where is your hope? A judge, like Caesar's wife should be above suspicion . . . We have suffered a grievous wrong, and an outrage has been put upon our city. Our officials have suffered a great indignity by being put under arrest. Our judges are our servants, paid to do our bidding and their duty.*[50]

Reverend Pedley had got it all wrong; Justice Crease would do nobody's bidding, and he would have been outraged at the minister's intensity. The Reverend Maxwell also further exacerbated the citizens of Victoria with his fiery sermons about "evil dignitaries."[51]

Above the clamour, and before the accused, Justice Crease calmly gave his ruling. He found Mayor Cope, City Solicitor Hamersley, and City Health Inspector Huntley guilty of contempt. "They have taken upon themselves Dominion duties and they have infringed upon the Dominion right of quarantine."[52] He hoped his ruling would end in his jurisdiction, and the case would not be dragged through federal courts. Crease also said that although the mayor and his council's actions were clearly illegal, they had acted with the welfare of Vancouver citizens in mind. Then, looking directly at Hamersley, he added, "They have been ill-advised . . . and I say that advisedly . . . erroneously advised."[53] The good judge blamed the lawyers. He ordered the injunction to be obeyed; handed Cope, Hamersley, and Huntley court costs; and set them free. Coming from Victoria was no longer an offence punishable by prison sentence.

The end of the smallpox wars also had an ironic twist. When the chastened mayor and his aides returned to Vancouver on the steamer *Comox*, they were forbidden to land. The notorious bylaw they had wrought had not yet been rescinded by city council. "A meeting was hastily convened on the dockside with the Mayor presiding from the deck of the ship."[54] Unfortunately, the dockside aldermen suddenly forgot their loyalties, believing that the three might have become infected while in Victoria and again put their beloved city at risk. They promptly adjourned and disembarked. Open-mouthed, Cope and his cohorts were stuck onboard just yards from shore.

• Was the isolated mayor, like Coleridge's ancient mariner, forced to tell his tale, "with long grey beard and glittering eye," to anyone who could be accosted long into the future? Not quite. The next morning, the Vancouver aldermen had a change of heart. They returned to the wharf and had the bylaw officially struck down. Ruffled and unsure what to think, Mayor Cope and his uneasy advisors crossed the gangplank and went home.

The whole affair was disastrous for British Columbians. Victoria recorded 112 cases of smallpox and 22 deaths. Vancouver recorded 19 cases and at least 9 deaths. Other infected coastal cities added 19 more cases and brought the total number to 150, with at least 30 deaths.[55] Fear, pomposity, and litigation had divided the citizens of Vancouver and Victoria. Those suffering personal losses over the smallpox epidemic endured far more. But the real culprit had, at last, been identified. The Albert Head Quarantine Station had a lot to answer for that dreadful summer of 1892, and barely two months later, the assault against it began in earnest.

Parry Bay Showing William Head and Albert Head •••

ALBERT HEAD
QUARANTINE STATION
Witty's Lagoon
Ⓐ

Witty's Beach

To Victoria

Taylor Beach

Weir's Beach
Ⓒ
Parry Bay

FIRST
NATIONS
LANDS
Ⓔ

WILLIAM HEAD
QUARANTINE STATION
Ⓑ

Pedder Bay

Becher Bay

Rocky Point

Eemdyk Passage

Ⓓ

BENTINCK ISLAND
LEPER COLONY
Ⓕ

Whirl Bay

Race Passage

Race Rocks

N
0 ———— 1
nautical miles

A. Albert Head Original Quarantine Station
B. William Head Quarantine Station
C. World War II Army Camp
D. Settlement at Anchorage
E. First Nations Lands
F. Bentinck Island Leper Colony

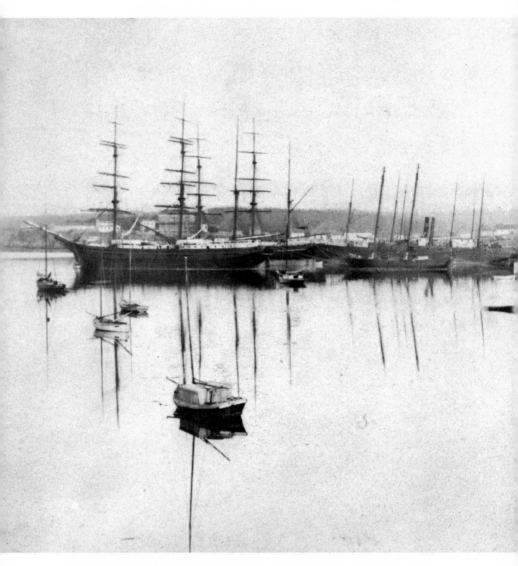

Those on the *Prince Alfred* in 1872 would have seen this view of Victoria Harbour. Note the customs house at the foot of Broughton Street.

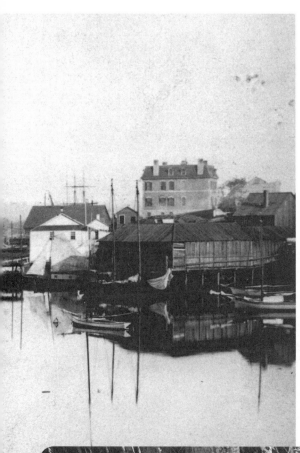

Hidden by Camus flowers
and tall grasses for
much of the year, a more
fortunate five-year-old
(Rowan Chow) stands
beside Bertha Whitney's
memorial stone in 2012.

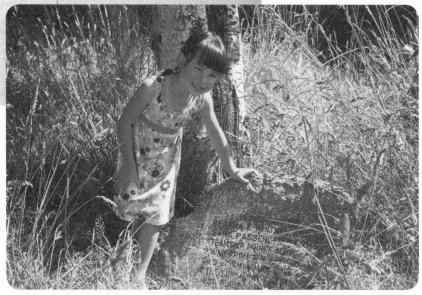

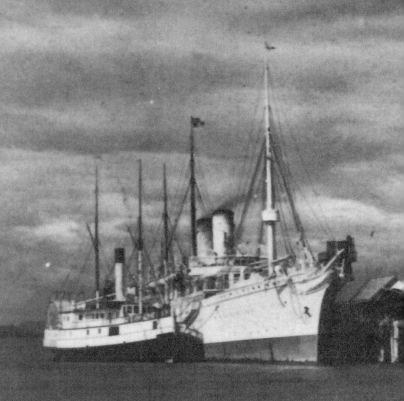

Bertha Whitney died thirty years before the *Empress of India* and the *Princess Louise* were directed to the William Head Quarantine Station wharf in 1901. METCHOSIN SCHOOL MUSEUM

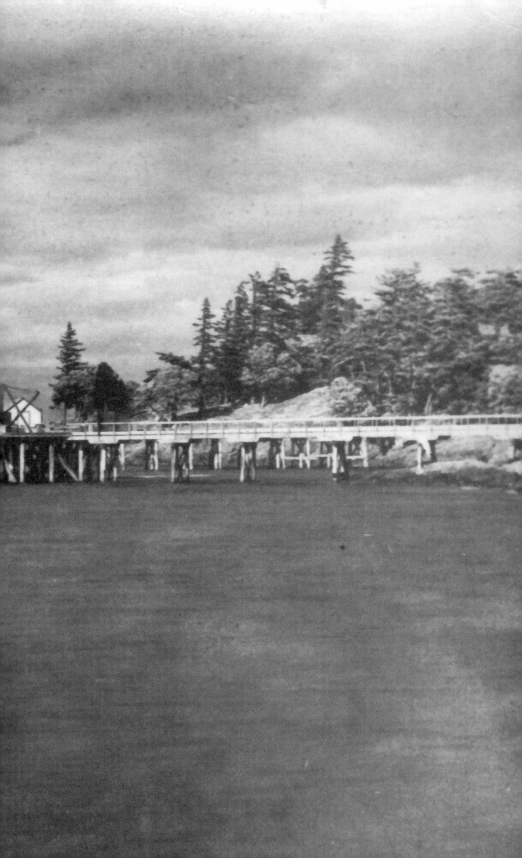

This ship, the *Empress of Japan*, carried the microbes that began the smallpox wars of 1889–92. METCHOSIN SCHOOL MUSEUM

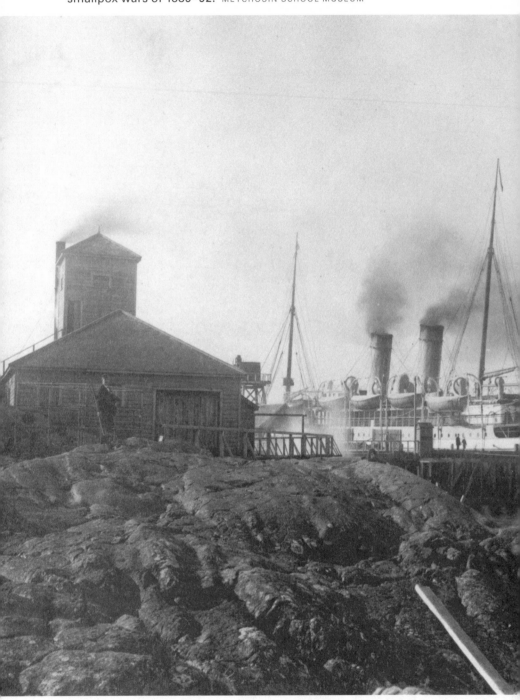

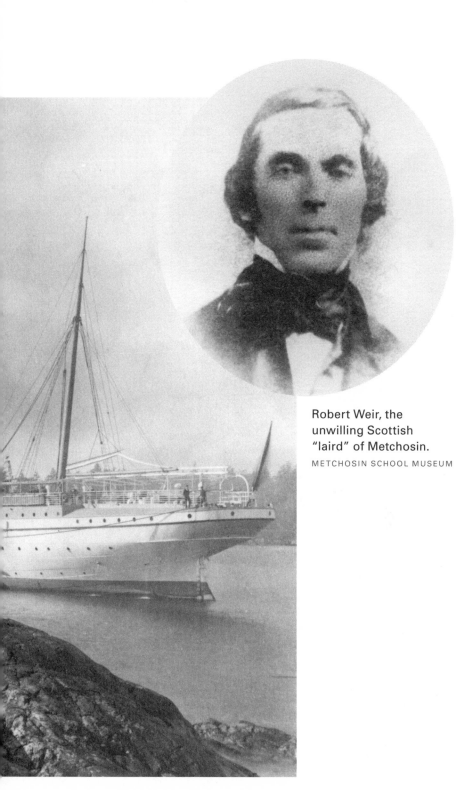

Robert Weir, the
unwilling Scottish
"laird" of Metchosin.
METCHOSIN SCHOOL MUSEUM

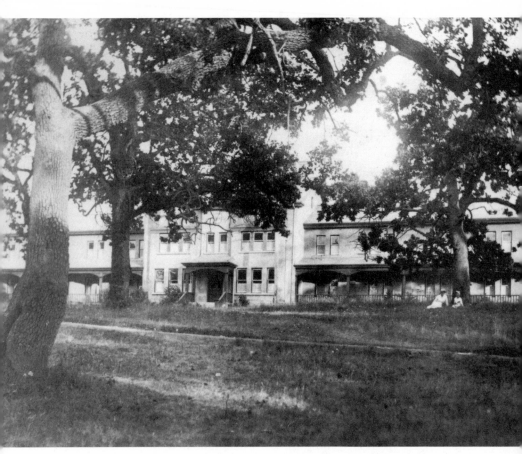

First-class hospital and first-class detention building, 1930s.

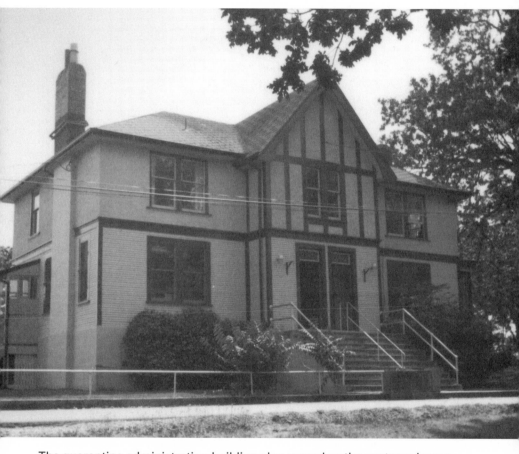

The quarantine administration building also served as the customs house for a time. METCHOSIN SCHOOL MUSEUM

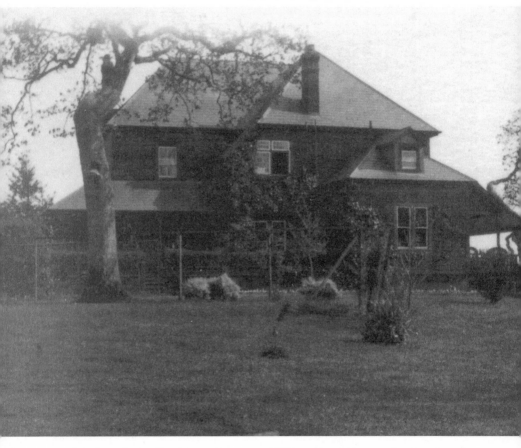

Chief medical officer's residence at William Head Quarantine Station, circa 1940s. CITY OF VICTORIA ARCHIVES, M09068

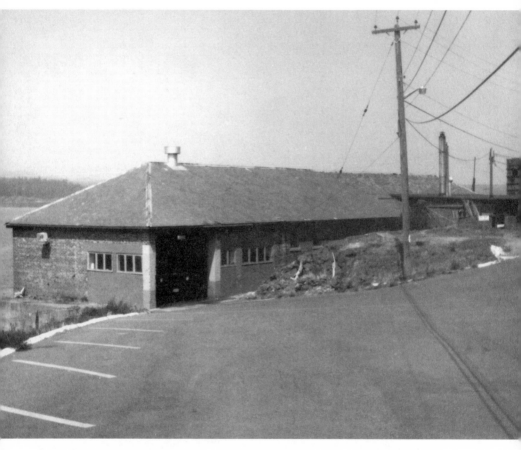

Fumigation building along the wharf. METCHOSIN SCHOOL MUSEUM

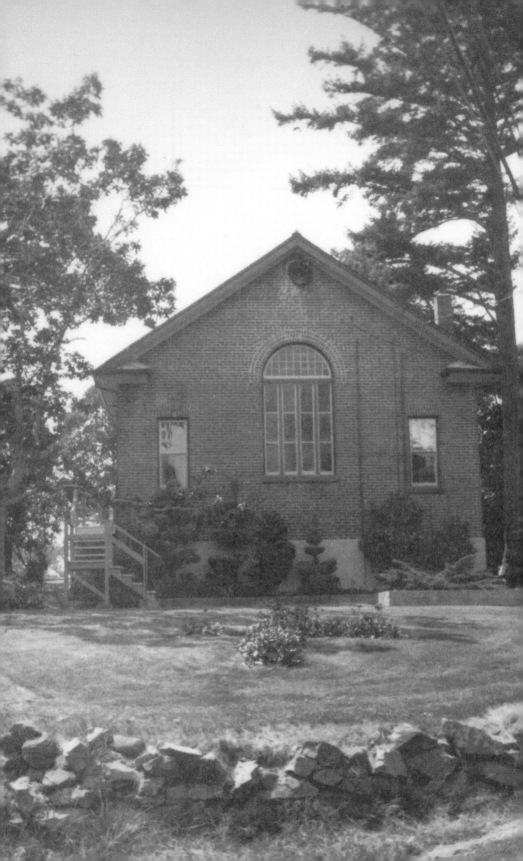

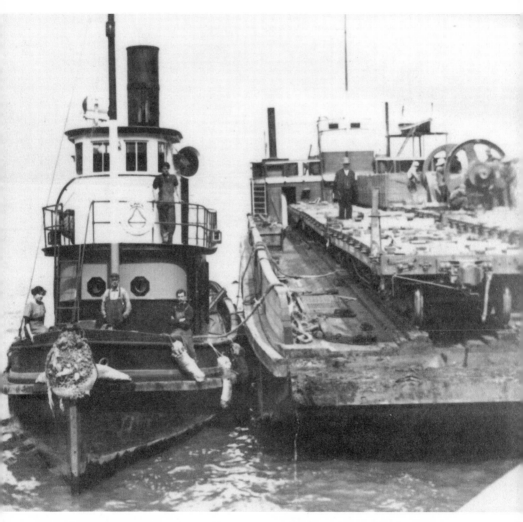

above The *Earle* delivered medical officers to ships in the often boisterous
Strait of Juan de Fuca. METCHOSIN SCHOOL MUSEUM

opposite Quarantine station school and chapel, circa 1930s.
METCHOSIN SCHOOL MUSEUM

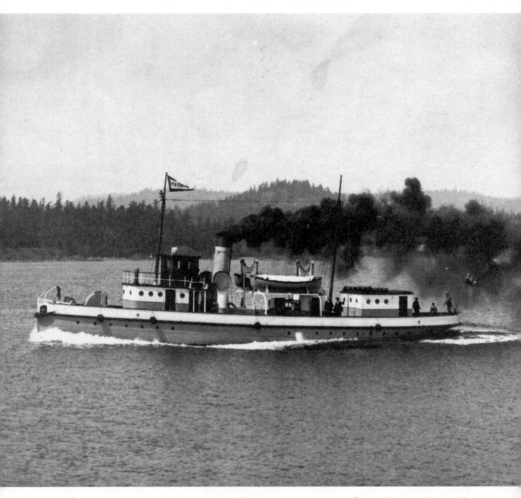

Quarantine inspection vessel *Madge* steaming out from the station with medical officers and customs officials on board. METCHOSIN SCHOOL MUSEUM

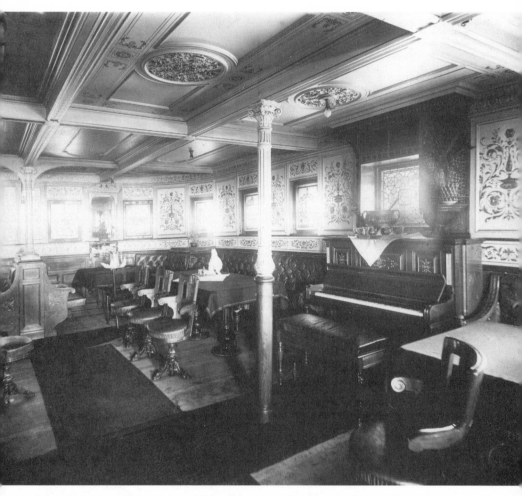

The first-class dining salon of the *Empress of Japan*—a far cry from the less-than-luxurious facilities at William Head. VANCOUVER MARITIME MUSEUM

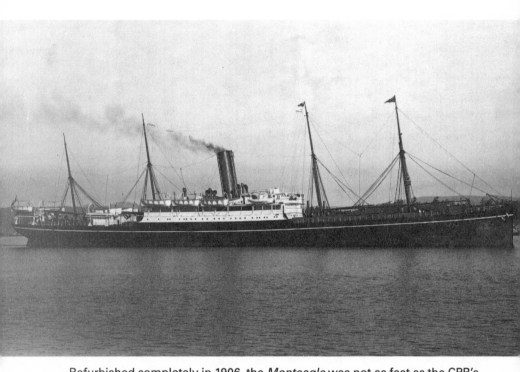

Refurbished completely in 1906, the *Monteagle* was not as fast as the CPR's "white empresses," but she was luxurious. VANCOUVER MARITIME MUSEUM

CHAPTER 4 // OMISSIONS, COMMISSIONS, AND CLOSURE

Will the weasel lie down with the snowshoe hare,
in the calm and peaceable kingdom?
Will the wolverine cease to rend and tear,
in the calm and peaceable kingdom?
Will the children feed grass to the grizzly bear,
in the calm and peaceable kingdom?

—David Helwig, "One Step from an Old Dance"[1]

I f he was anything, William Ellison was a man of principle. He had witnessed the anguish and hostility of slum dwellers in East London and the destitute of the rat-infested port cities of India. As rector of a small rural church west of Victoria, his values would be tested. In Metchosin, Ellison found a hugely dysfunctional institution. The Albert Head Quarantine Station had been operational for just over five years when Ellison arrived at St. Mary's Anglican Church in 1892. Yet the conditions at the station and its treatment of quarantined detainees had deteriorated to the point where those in the nearby village feared that violence might erupt at any moment. At the station, Reverend Ellison found facilities unfit for habitation, an indifferent staff, and hungry detainees. He was so shocked at the potential for violence that this gentle man of God stated publicly that he seriously considered packing a gun.

Reverend Ellison's charges against the Albert Head Quarantine Station stood at the end point of a long public outcry that brought the place to its knees.

William George Hollingsworth Ellison was bound to become a minister. He was born in the prosperous royalist city of Lichfield, Staffordshire, whose famous Gothic cathedral had been damaged by parliamentarians during the Civil War. As a child in 1867, William saw the old cathedral restored to its former elegance. He marvelled at its three eccentric spires and loved the sound of its recast bells as they pealed across a diocese that stretched from the green hills of Shropshire to the Black Country of the West Midlands.

By the time William was an adolescent, the Anglican Church was in his blood. He would become one of those "Muscular Christians" inspired by the missionary David Livingstone, whose exploits were so much a part of nineteenth-century church life. Like many others of his time, he planned to serve in the colonies doing "good works" for the Lord, then return home to a safe country parish in the rolling, green hills of his youth.

By 1883, he was working as a priest in a parish in East London. By 1890, he was chaplain in Mumbai, which had become the centre of trade between India and the rest of the world as silk, muslin, rice, onyx, tobacco, and cotton moved to Mecca, Basra, Cape Town, Cadiz, and London. Here, Portuguese, Mughals, and British intermingled and secretly married—and here, too, under a mélange of exotic tongues, beliefs, and castes, merchant seamen often found themselves adrift. For them, Ellison founded a seaman's institute and organized an emigration society for India's truly destitute. It was in Mumbai that he began a lifelong study of comparative religions.

In 1892, Reverend Ellison was posted as a "missionary clergyman" to St. Mary's Anglican Church in Metchosin, British Columbia. India had made him wiser and bolder. He was the first Anglican churchman in British Columbia to perform a marriage between a white man and a Chinese woman, and he allowed St. Mary's Anglican Church to be used for the burial service of a Catholic priest. Later Ellison would speak out vehemently against the British in the Boer War.

At the Albert Head Quarantine Station, Ellison found an inordinate number of Chinese detainees, and discovered that their incarceration and treatment was disproportionately more severe than that of others. He had seen this kind of racism before and loathed it. In a letter to the *Colonist* in March 1893, he wrote,

I found a poor Japanese [Chinese?] digging for clams on the foreshore outside the quarantine limits at Albert Head. He said he and his companions had been ten weeks in quarantine, and, during the last fortnight, they had been kept so short of food they had to hunt for clams and seaweed.

My neighbor tells me they have cleaned him out . . . and have generally foraged all over the neighborhood. Those Japs [Chinese], I was given to understand, were in quarantine. If so, it must be a ghastly joke to have them wandering around living on what they can pick up in the neighborhood.[2]

Ellison believed that someone at Albert Head was "squandering the cash" intended for the purchase of food for Chinese detainees. He discovered that they alone were forced to earn their meagre nourishment by chopping firewood. This treatment, he charged, was against the law. Ellison also witnessed chronic retching and lashed out against the station's lack of fresh water. It was a major defect that had plagued Albert Head from the beginning. He claimed that the little potable water was brackish, "uncertain," and wholly inappropriate for a medical facility. Experiencing Metchosin's frequent winter windstorms, he saw trees lying across the station's waterline, and noted, "since a tree has fallen and uprooted the line, the only water to be got [for Albert Head] was from a neighbouring cattle pond, from which buckets are taken daily."[3]

Metchosin settlers read Ellison's letter with interest, and told him of their own fears of the ravenous, marauding, and perhaps contagious detainees. Within a short time, he became the spokesman for the citizens of his parish. "I am afraid that if any large number of Orientals are placed in quarantine at Albert Head without a more efficient guard, we may be attacked by a starving herd of hungry men . . . I am looking to my guns in case of emergency."[4]

Ellison made it patently clear that the conditions at the facility were completely untenable and that something needed to be done urgently. By March 1893, no one disagreed. He wrote, "The Albert Head Quarantine Station was, for as long as I could remember, considered little more than a joke."[5]

THE "JOKE" HAD BEGUN to unravel just six months before when a reporter for the *British Colonist* made his way into the station and decided to tell all. His searing denunciation of the quarantine facility alerted Victoria citizens to the dark fact that the province still had no institutional means of preventing incoming contagion. Albert Head was no bulwark against infectious disease, and being "cleared" simply meant the contagious could run amok. The article stated:

> [The station] is destitute of all the appliances which a quarantine station should have. It is difficult to approach, both by sea and land. It has no wharf to accommodate craft of any kind. The building could afford a rude shelter for a few people for only a very short time. They could not be lodged properly and they could not be fed. There are no conveniences for cooking in anything like a large scale, and the water supply is uncertain and scanty. To make matters worse, the station has no kind of communication with the capital or other inhabited parts of the province. It is certainly isolated, but its isolation is the isolation of desolation.
>
> Neither the people of the Dominion, nor the people of this province should, for one moment, shut their eyes to the fact that as regards the diseases which the quarantine station is established to guard against, the Pacific Coast of the Dominion is perfectly defenceless.[6]

Others knew long before that the problems at Albert Head were not limited solely to its facilities; the real issue was the competence of its staff. By July 1892, the people of Victoria had been pushed to the limit. They had suffered a blockade, an epidemic, violence, and the fury of litigation. On the evening of July 20, 1892, Mayor Robert Beaven set aside his council's usual agenda and moved on to a report placed before them. The report was written by Dr. M.S. Wade, the provincial health officer, who had spent considerable time observing conditions and practices at Albert Head that spring. It was a complete condemnation of those who worked at the quarantine station.

Dr. Wade's report noted that many smallpox sufferers were removed from Albert Head to a municipal hospital in Victoria as Ottawa continued to treat the federal west coast facility with its usual niggling neglect. The salaries of seven nurses who worked at the station had to be paid for by the City, and two additional nurses were privately subcontracted. Of the seven, only two, Mr. Tite and Mr. Blake, had any experience in infectious disease control. Wade also recorded that the wives of two detained patients were allowed to mingle freely with others throughout the station while supposedly nursing their sick husbands.

Then came the bombshell: Nurse Joseph Harrison, manager of a unit, was "thoroughly incapable, negligent, and inefficient, was drunk most of the time and was, at the time, living in a tent on-site with the wife of one of the patients."[7] Overseeing physicians, Victoria health officers Dr. Crompton and Dr. Rundle Nelson, who should have exercised some clout, made only three visits in a period of one month.

The details of other such practices abounded. Wade noted that medical supplies arrived only intermittently, and suppliers readily intermingled with nurses and patients alike. The drinking water, though now being delivered, was done so in unregulated vinegar, wine, or whiskey casks, which created a disagreeable flavour. When two cases of whiskey were delivered to the station, they lasted only a few days.[8] Even worse, the food delivery was sporadic, its quality poor, and its preparation "was being done at irregular hours by anyone able to do it."[9]

Medical records spoke for themselves. In May, just prior to the summer epidemic, fifteen cases of smallpox had been quarantined from inbound ships; five of those patients became seriously ill, and three died. The graves of the dead were so shallow, Dr. Wade charged, that pathogens from a decaying corpse were close enough to the surface to pose an active danger to public health. In short, the Albert Head Quarantine Station was in complete shambles. According to Wade, the man responsible was Dr. Charles Milne, Victoria's municipal health officer.

In the Victoria council chambers, Dr. Wade's report was met with a surfeit of uncomfortable coughing. Finally, Councillor Lovell said that those in charge of the place "had no doubt proved themselves negligent and unfit for their position."[10] He believed, however, that Dr. Milne should at least be given the opportunity to respond.

Mayor Beaven summoned Dr. Milne, who stated outright that the foodstuffs and other supplies were sufficient and in good supply. Then he wavered. He admitted that the Victoria unit at the quarantine station was overstaffed, and nurse Harrison, being "dictatorial and overbearing," had been fired. Of the widespread whiskey consumption, Milne said he knew nothing, but admitted that *he* had ordered two bottles of brandy as a stimulant for some patients. He accepted that the water "may have been tainted," and the disinfectant showers needed a "slight improvement," but argued that, overall, Albert Head's facilities were as good as others in the city. Nonplussed, he rejected Dr. Wade's report, stating "it was merely made on hearsay or founded on imagination."[11]

Soon after, Dr. Wade's report was leaked to the newspapers, and several of the implicated defended themselves through the press. Charles Tite, a male nurse with supposed experience in smallpox treatment, wrote, "Gentlemen—I wish to say that much of Dr. Wade's report is untrue. I was not intoxicated at Albert Head, nor was Harrison. The remarks regarding the Woman and myself are untrue. Five bottles of whiskey were used in sponging Mr. Western . . ."[12]

Besides admitting to a most unorthodox medical treatment, and a terrible misuse of good whiskey, Nurse Tite was lying. He resigned his position when three patients, Fred Foster, Edward Sexton, and T.L. Baron, published their reply, which read: "We desire to say that Mr. Tite was for the most of his time, intoxicated as was also Mr. Harrison, and we were treated in a manner that was shameful. We had breakfast when we could get it; lunch when the nurses were sober, and dinner when we could get it."[13]

The bottom fell further out of Dr. Milne's universe when a letter from Mr. Poole, the administrative officer in charge of the Albert Head Quarantine Station, published a note supporting Dr. Wade's report:

M.S. WADE, ESQ., MD,

Dear Sir; With regard to what took place down here, I am prepared to swear to your report as being correct in every particular, but I do not like to write for publication in the papers.

Your obedient servant, Walter Poole[14]

Mayor Beaven acted quickly. He had Dr. Milne removed from all responsibilities connected with smallpox control at the Albert Head Quarantine Station. At the end of July 1892, Victoria citizens read of a smallpox outbreak in Gretna, a small village in southern Manitoba. Miss Calder, a missionary from Winnipeg, caught the disease while visiting the Chinese of the village to evangelize, and went on to infect other members of the hamlet. The Chinese had avoided detection at Albert Head.

On August 10, Vancouver health officer Joseph Huntley wrote to provincial health officer Dr. J.C. Davie, revealing how nineteen cases of smallpox in Vancouver could be traced to the April 17 inbound voyage of the *Empress of Japan*. He said, "I have not the least doubt that nearly, if not quite all, the cases you have had in Victoria might be traced to this same, most prolific source."[15] Huntley believed the sources were Chinese steerage passengers from the *Empress* who "were not kept under surveillance for the requisite length of time at the [Albert Head] station, but were discharged."[16] Mr. Huntley was frustrated with the laxity at Albert Head and demanded that the needless spread of infectious disease receive "urgent attention."

Premier Davie received Huntley's letter and promptly telegraphed Ottawa:

THE MINISTER OF MARINE AND FISHERIES, OTTAWA— AUG. 25, 1892. *This Government proposes appointing a Commission to enquire into the causes which led to the recent outbreak of smallpox in this Province, and best means of preventing recurrence of smallpox and introduction of other epidemic and endemic diseases.*

We propose appoint Chief Justice Begbie and two competent medical men. Facts point to introduction of smallpox by Canadian Pacific steamers from Asiatic ports, and responsibility resting with Dominion

Government, to whom is entrusted the promulgation and enforcement of quarantine regulations.

Will Dominion Government join in the Commission and name one of the Commissioners so as to preserve and collect the evidence?

No time is to be lost.

—THEODORE DAVIE, PREMIER[17]

Ottawa flatly refused to participate in the commission because they knew that they could be financially liable if found culpable. Unfazed by Ottawa's rejection, British Columbia decided to move ahead, and on October 6, 1892, the province ordered a commission to inquire into the past summer's epidemic of smallpox. Chief Justice Matthew Begbie and Dr. Alex E. Praeger were appointed commissioners. Their report would demand that Ottawa make financial reparations for the "damage done by lax administration, and seek a committed financial base for future epidemics should they arise again."[18] Absent or not, the Canadian government was going to be shamed into doing what federal law required—fix the horror at Albert Head.

Begbie and Praeger were guided by two questions. They wanted to know the details of how smallpox arrived in the province that summer and how it spread so quickly.

In three months, the commission called fifty-six witnesses. Its findings, submitted in February 20, 1893, pointed to administrative irregularities, financial improprieties, lax enforcement of existing quarantine regulations, and very bad luck.

Still piqued by his loss of status, Dr. Milne testified that up to July 1892, "there had been no case here [in Vancouver] for four or five years."[19] Dr. MacNaughton-Jones, chief medical officer at the Albert Head Quarantine Station, recalled the December 1891 case of Mrs. Livingstone. Mr. Huntley recollected several similar cases that occurred in Vancouver the year before. Dr. Aitkins reminded the commission of Aboriginal epidemics in the 1860s, and stated "the province was never clear from it."[20] Indeed, since Bertha Whitney's arrival in 1872 and the ensuing surge in shipping soon after, smallpox outbreaks persisted. Worse, quarantine regulations, which the *Colonist* explained were "framed originally for Atlantic and

St. Lawrence ports, and not at all suited to the Pacific province,"[21] remained unchanged. Clearly, Dr. Milne was out of touch.

Justice Begbie and Dr. Praeger recorded not only that cases of smallpox went unnoticed by medical officers but also that many were misdiagnosed. Victoria citizen Fred Wright, who did *not* have smallpox, was mistakenly sent to the smallpox unit at Royal Jubilee Hospital, while David Smith, who *did* have smallpox, was not quarantined at the facility because a newly appointed Victoria health officer thought he had something else. Begbie and Praeger noted that such mix-ups were due to the distasteful conditions of quarantine stations and to "government instructions having a tendency to laxity . . . All measures of quarantine were so damaging to individuals and commerce that the public would simply not tolerate anything but the most necessary precautions."[22]

The real worth of the 1892 commission lay in its tracking of the movements of smallpox carriers that fateful summer of 1892 and its certainty that the epidemic began with the inattentiveness of quarantine officers at Albert Head. Vancouver health officer Joseph Huntley had tracked the whereabouts of undetected smallpox carriers across Georgia Strait. His analysis stands as a landmark in epidemiological sleuthing in British Columbia, and his thoroughness marked him as an investigator of groundbreaking ability. His knowledge was critical to the commission's understanding of other testimony, and it bears relating.

In 1892, Harry Farrar worked as a longshoreman and sometimes deckhand on the Canadian Pacific Navigation Company steamer *Yosemite*. Often, he helped load and unload cargo from the CPN ships *Yosemite* and *Islander* at their Victoria wharf. On May 25, while living on Herald Street in Victoria, Farrar fell ill. Dr. Helmcken saw Farrar and sent him to the Royal Jubilee Hospital with a "suspected bladder complaint."[23] There, Dr. Richardson diagnosed him with smallpox and refused to admit him. Dr. Richardson then sent Farrar to see Dr. Milne, the Victoria health officer. Milne concurred with Richardson's diagnosis, and sent Farrar away under a "stay-at-home" order.

Harry Farrar's illness progressed. While at home, he was visited by many friends, including a Mr. Fitzpatrick, who stayed overnight. A few days later, Farrar noticed red spots on his wrists and demanded to be taken to the Albert Head Quarantine Station by a hackman (carriage driver) whom he knew personally. At Albert Head, Farrar and his driver were placed under quarantine.

Strangely, while isolated at Albert Head, Farrar was visited several more times by his friends from Victoria. Where exactly these friends went after they left is unknown; their stories were never heard by the commission.

It became known that a young child living close to Harry Farrar, at Louis College on Pandora Street, contracted smallpox at the end of June. City health inspectors quarantined the college and placed a guard at the gates. Fortunately the child's case was mild, and "when she recovered the bedding and such like were burned and all the clothing and the rooms as well, were disinfected."[24] Another child, also living close by on Pandora Street, was found to have caught the disease as well. She was not quarantined. Then, on July 4, two more children, Annie Hamilton and Georgina Campbell, who lived at the nearby refuge home, developed smallpox. Although the refuge home was quarantined and both cases treated on-site, Annie Hamilton died of the disease.

The spread of smallpox among Victoria's children during the summer holidays that year gave cause for alarm. Dr. Milne testified that as soon as a case of childhood smallpox was reported to him, "he had the house quarantined."[25] He recounted the case of F.C. McWinn's young son: "When the case was reported to me on Friday [July 8], the Clarence Hotel where the child lived with his parents, was quarantined by noon on Saturday."[26] Yet, earlier testimony revealed that the child was removed from the Clarence Hotel under Dr. Milne's personal supervision on Wednesday night (July 6), and the Clarence Hotel was only sealed after a lapse of three days. The commissioners believed that this three-day lapse in the containment of the disease was a dangerously long time. Mayor Beaven decried Milne's delayed "stay-at-home quarantine," and in consequence constructed a special smallpox-only unit on the grounds of the Royal Jubilee Hospital, away from the Albert Head Quarantine Station.

Harry Farrar's case of smallpox turned out to be mild, but those at the hearings soon understood that even the mildest case of smallpox could result in a deadly condition in others. By July 12, just two weeks into summer, there were seventeen active cases of smallpox scattered throughout the city.[27]

As the number of cases steadily increased, a pattern began to emerge. Mr. Barrows, who lived on Pandora Street close to the infected children's homes, also became ill. Mr. Huntley revealed that Mr. Barrows had travelled to Vancouver in early June for the annual Foresters' Excursion Picnic and while there had visited two friends, Mr. Marsh and Mr. Williams. Huntley followed Marsh's trail and discovered that within the same week he had visited another Vancouver resident, a Mrs. Bibby. Mr. Huntley showed that Mrs. Bibby was already ill with smallpox in mid-May. Barrows remained in Vancouver for a month after the Foresters' picnic, and returned to Victoria on July 16 with Marsh and Williams on the *Islander*.

Because of the relative isolation of Mr. Barrows's Pandora Street address, it was first believed that he became infected through the schoolchildren in his neighbourhood. After Mr. Huntley's testimony, however, it was believed he had caught the disease from Marsh or Williams, his companions in Vancouver, one of whom had close contact with Mrs. Bibby. The circle had been closed. The origin of the smallpox epidemic was traced "to the date of the Foresters' picnic to Vancouver City"[28] and to the return to Victoria of infected carriers on July 16. The shock came when the commissioners heard Huntley's account of the nefarious sojourns of Mrs. Bibby.

In the meantime, the Clarence Hotel in Victoria had been placed under quarantine, and several patients, all diagnosed with smallpox, were confined to their rooms. The quarantine regulations at the Clarence Hotel were applied when many of those infected were absent and hence prohibited from re-entering the premises. Those who were first infected had been allowed to wander freely on the streets, becoming sicker by the minute, when they should never have been allowed to leave in the first place. When the quarantine order came down and they were not allowed back in, the "homeless" infected carriers put the whole city at risk.

The testimony of Fred Phillips, a hackman who lived at the Clarence Hotel, gave the farce an even more bizarre twist. On July 8, just before the quarantine order took effect, Phillips was asked to take a Mr. Sandy

Williams on a recreational drive into the country. Upon calling at Williams's Broad Street address on Saturday morning, he discovered that the gentleman had smallpox. Phillips refused his services and left. Later that weekend, Phillips suffered severe back pains and visited Dr. Milne, who told him he had developed "cold in the kidneys"[29] and to go home. He did, but he was prevented from entering his rooms as the quarantine order had taken effect in his absence. Fred Phillips "was driven out of the very place in which he ought to have been confined, and went and slept instead at the Delmonico Hotel."[30] A day later, still suffering, Phillips drove over to the Royal Jubilee Hospital, where he was refused entry, "as there was no accommodation." That night he slept in a tent. On Tuesday, complete with a rash and now very ill, Mr. Phillips was diagnosed with smallpox.

Arthur B. Monkhouse was a night telegrapher with the District Telegraph Company and he too roomed at the Clarence Hotel. On Thursday, July 5, he went to bed ill. On Thursday, he was visited by Dr. Sproule, who assured him "that he had *not* got the smallpox."[31] That Friday, July 8, his friends from the company office visited him in his room. By Saturday morning, a rash had broken out, but as Dr. Sproule did not make a return visit, Arthur Monkhouse went out for a walk. He went to Russell's Barber Shop for a bath and a shave and visited the company office, where a friend advised him to see Dr. Milne. Dr. Milne confirmed that he had smallpox and told him to go home. By the time he returned, the Clarence Hotel had been placed under quarantine and he was forbidden entry, so he returned to Dr. Milne who gave him written authority to retrace his contagious steps home through Victoria's streets yet again.

The role of the Clarence Hotel in the spread of Victoria's smallpox epidemic became even more incredible with the story of Mr. and Mrs. Niles. At the time of the epidemic, the couple lived above Eckhart's Grocery, next door to the Clarence Hotel. A dressmaker, Mrs. Niles asserted that though smallpox had killed her husband, it had *nothing* to do with a parcel of dresses that she had sent out to be altered by her seamstress, Miss Bull, who had also caught smallpox. Did she catch it from Mr. Niles, from the infected clothing, or from Clarence Hotel residents who often visited

Eckhart's Grocery next door? Had she become a carrier? The furtive and silent epidemic continued to spread like frost on glass.

The key to this whole infectious efflorescence was traced to the April 17, 1892, arrival of the *Empress of Japan* from Yokohama, which had arrived off Albert Head en route to Vancouver. Captain Lee and the ship's surgeon, Dr. Temple, raised some eyebrows when they gave testimony suggesting that Dr. MacNaughton-Jones was lax in his medical inspection of the ship. Evidence from the ship's log noted that the *Empress* "dropped anchor off Victoria at 6:07 p.m., and she received a letter of pratique [clearance] at 6:30 p.m. . . . barely twenty-three minutes later."[32] Considering that there were some 516 Chinese steerage passengers on board, this meant that over 20 suspect Chinese passengers would have had to have been examined and assessed for infectious disease each and every minute of that time. Moreover, Lee and Temple stated that Dr. MacNaughton-Jones was not on board during the whole inspection. Dr. MacNaughton-Jones denied the charges.

When the *Empress of Japan* arrived in Vancouver, Mr. Huntley discovered a single case of smallpox, that of a Chinese passenger in steerage.[33] At that point, Huntley ordered all 516 passengers and the ship itself back to the Albert Head Quarantine Station. The infected man was placed in the station hospital, while the others were held in the so-called Chinese detention quarters.

Official quarantine regulations at the time demanded that patients under observation be watched for nine days from an outbreak. The hospitalized Chinese patient had not shown any progressive symptoms at the time of his quarantine, so he and his countrymen were released eight days later.[34] Of the 516 released, 278 remained in Victoria. On April 27, two days later, 238 Chinese boarded the *Islander,* bound for Vancouver. Mr. Farrar would have been on the Victoria wharf that day.

While there was no direct evidence presented at the enquiry that other cases had developed among Chinese passengers, it became known that two of them had travelled at the end of April to Gretna, Manitoba, where a young missionary nurse and others in the village were in for the shock of their lives.

Two officials, Mr. Reid and Mr. Hyde, worked at the Vancouver Customs House, where the Chinese from the *Empress of Japan* were processed after their arrival in Vancouver. Both caught the disease and, in turn, spread it to their friend, a Mr. Stott, and to his friend, Mr. Leask, who lived in an old cabin on the seashore of Burrard Inlet. Mr. Barnett, a ticket agent for the CPR in Vancouver, provided tickets for the two Gretna-bound Chinese passengers on the April 30 transcontinental train. Barnett too fell ill.

Two longshoremen named Mr. Harrington and Mr. Gillick worked on the CPR wharves in Vancouver and constantly handled baggage from the steamers *Islander* and *Yosemite*. Both Harrington and Gillick were stricken. Though locked out of Vancouver, the ships were never fumigated.

The pièce de résistance came when Mr. Huntley traced the movements of Mrs. Bibby. He discovered that she and a male companion, Tupper Thompson, had both been on that April 17 voyage of the *Empress of Japan*. She had not been detained at the Albert Head Quarantine Station but had proceeded directly to the mainland along with those Chinese passengers who had been summarily released. Three weeks later, Mr. Huntley had found Mrs. Bibby gravely ill in a house of ill repute on Dupont Street in Vancouver. Mr. Marsh had visited this popular prostitute at exactly the time when she was most contagious. She, Tupper Thompson, and most of her clients died of smallpox.

The commission had uncovered the source and track of the summer epidemic of smallpox in Victoria and Vancouver in 1892. It began, as Mr. Huntley rightly believed, with one known case of a Chinese passenger who was diagnosed with smallpox on April 17. He had spread it to Mrs. Bibby and seven others in Vancouver (Reid, Hyde, Stott, Laesk, Barnett, Harrison, and Gillick). Mrs. Bibby then passed the disease on to Marsh, who, along with Williams and Barrows, carried the disease back to Vancouver Island. Once in Victoria, it blossomed among the white population, beginning with residents at the ill-fated Clarence Hotel.

The commission decided that Harry Farrar, the Victoria longshoreman, most likely caught smallpox from the Chinese on the *Empress of Japan* who milled about the Victoria wharves after being prematurely released from the Albert Head Quarantine Station on April 27.

The reason the smallpox epidemic spread so quickly throughout Victoria and Vancouver that summer, they believed, was due to medical officers lacking information about the disease, and their lax and inconsistent manner of upholding quarantine regulations. Newly appointed provincial health officer Dr. Davie would soon lay down the law and instate new quarantine regulations.[35]

The commission was not allowed to lay blame, but it censured Dr. Milne. They reiterated that the health of all citizens depended upon a strong working relationship between provincial and municipal agents. The report noted, "And the want of accord between the views of the Provincial Health Officer and the Municipal Officer made the suspension of the latter, an absolute necessity, in order to secure obedience to the Provincial Regulations."[36] Given the severity of the epidemic, Dr. Milne was lucky not to have been thrown out of the profession.

Victoria's decision to use part of the Albert Head Quarantine Station during the epidemic was soundly condemned by the report. The commissioners cited its distance from Victoria, lack of proper facilities, and improperly trained personnel—not to mention an overall laxity—which rendered it useless as a treatment facility. In its recommendations, the commission did not mince words, and its list of objectives to "invert all conditions" that had lead to the epidemic of 1892 were far-reaching:

- That all health districts (municipalities) in British Columbia establish two separate quarantine facilities: one a hospital with a resident physician to treat already developed cases of smallpox, and the other a separate "suspect station" in which all persons having contact with the ill would be held.
- That an isolation hospital be established on Deadman's Island in Vancouver and Poplar Island in New Westminster, equipped with "proper air filters," making them "safer in even the most crowded cities."[37]
- That the provincial health officer be given the right of removal, isolation, and treatment of person or persons suspected of having smallpox to an appropriate medical facility.

- That all municipalities in British Columbia no longer legislate bylaws affecting epidemics, and such legislation be entrusted only to the provincial health officer.
- That vaccination be made compulsory for all children before the age of three months, and be repeated at puberty.
- That all cases of infectious diseases be recorded and a register kept of all vaccinated citizens.
- That federal quarantine officers inspect all ships, cargo, crew, and passengers daily while under orders of quarantine at a federal station and such reinspection be done in during daylight.
- That fumigation of ships' cargoes be facilitated through a dioxide blast machine, and consumable foodstuffs personally inspected by a competent authority.
- That all ships' doctors be accredited and be made responsible to the provincial health officer.
- That costs of quarantine treatment *not* be "thrown entirely on the respective municipalities; but a proportion, at least, of such expenses should be borne by the Dominion of Canada."[38] The Dominion, however, should be invested with a voice in its management.
- That cremation of diseased victims of infectious disease be encouraged and bodies of victims not be allowed to leave the grounds of an isolation hospital.
- That the sanitation of public ways and drains be maintained by the regular removal of filth, and rigid inspection of all "unhealthy" trades and establishments occur with special attention afforded to tenements and lodging houses.
- That a municipality's water supply be secured from a body of water designated as a watershed and be free from the contamination of human or farm habitation.

• • •

ON THE EVENING OF Friday, January 6, 1893, the British Columbia Board of Trade held its quarterly meeting in Victoria and heard an earful. First, Victoria Member of Parliament E.G. Prior reported his struggle with Ottawa bureaucrats to uphold their responsibilities. He read out the deputy minister's response to his enquiry regarding securing clean, fresh water for Albert Head. "It is outrageous to pay $80 to get in water. You should be able to get enough rain water from the roof."[39] Prior then read the deputy's view of a proposed new salary of $40 per month for the station's caretakers. "Why they can get all the fish they want by getting into their canoe; they can get all the wood they want on the beach, and they are very well paid."[40] Ottawa was simply uninterested in its west coast quarantine obligations.

Then Mr. Cannon of Northern Steamship Lines presented his solutions to the Albert Head Quarantine debacle. He referred to the April 17, 1892, sailing of the *Empress of Japan* in which hundreds of Chinese were quarantined at Alberta Head all too briefly. "In fact a landing could not be effected as the so-called wharf was in a wretched condition. More, when the unfortunate men were finally put ashore they were without shelter or food, or any means of cooking."[41] As agent for other trans-Pacific shipping companies, Cannon reported that he had to send lumber to the station to erect a temporary shed for the Chinese. His own company, he told the startled crowd, was forced to pay for food for all the detained passengers, and even hire their guards. Cannon rightly argued, "all this should have been provided by the Dominion government."[42] When Cannon concluded, "if there were to be a repetition of this sort of thing, our vessels, as well as others, would be obliged to shun the port,"[43] many in the room knew that Seattle would drool at the prospect of more business.

Dr. MacNaughton-Jones stepped up to read parts of his December 1892 report to the federal minister of agriculture. Growing weary of Ottawa's silence and the station's deteriorating conditions, MacNaughton-Jones had said, "Albert Head is inadequate for its requirements."[44] He told the assembly the unfortunate story of Mrs. Livingstone, who had been quarantined at Albert Head in 1891. Of the quarters she was forced to occupy, she had reportedly said that "they were not fit for an Indian."[45]

The conservative-minded Board of Trade passed several resolutions urging Ottawa to make immediate changes at Albert Head. For some, sensing a loss of business, the communiqués were too mild. They mumbled about closing the Albert Head Quarantine Station completely.

What the Board of Trade didn't know was that Dr. MacNaughton-Jones had already begun similar discussions with the federal department of public works. On January 31, 1893, the federal minister of agriculture instructed the commander-in-chief of the Royal Naval Base in Esquimalt; Rear Admiral Hotham; Captain Devereaux, superintendent of the naval dry dock; and engineer Mr. Gamble of the Victoria Public Works Department to come to Ottawa to discuss the location for the establishment of a new, permanent Dominion quarantine station. Reverend Ellison's damning letter of March 13, 1893, about the "joke" that was Albert Head had made the widespread outrage of ordinary citizens patently clear. It was to become the impetus for the wheels of bureaucracy to move more quickly.

• • •

THE SHORT, TROUBLED LIFE of the Albert Head Quarantine Station ended in April 1893 when federal officials shut down the facility. There is a curious irony in its closing. The peninsula on which it stood was named after Prince Albert of Saxe-Coburg, Prince Consort, husband, and first cousin of Queen Victoria. Contemporary medical officials believed that Albert's untimely death was caused by another infectious contagion that had thus far avoided detection—typhoid.

CHAPTER 5 // SECOND WIND: A ROUSING GOOD GO

"When the hurlyburly's done, When the battle's lost and won."

—William Shakespeare, *Macbeth*, 1.1

obert Beaven was nobody's fool. Resolute and feisty, he was a natural politician. As finance minister in the Legislative Assembly in 1881, he seconded the motion to have British Columbia withdraw from Confederation. He had become so livid with Ottawa's reluctance to honour British Columbia's subsidy that he asked Princess Louise, the wife of Governor General John Campbell, the Marquess of Lorne, if she would become queen of an independent Vancouver Island. She declined.

Controversial to the last, Beaven got his values and fighting spirit from his father, a clergyman and professor of metaphysics. Robert graduated from Upper Canada College in 1858 and promptly left Ontario for adventure and gold in the Cariboo. He married, settled in Victoria, sold sewing machines, and bought real estate. In 1868, he joined Amor De Cosmos's Confederation League to save the province from privateers and was elected to the British Columbia legislature in 1871. He would become its longest-serving member.

Robert Beaven became premier of British Columbia in 1882, then leader of the official opposition in 1883, and was mayor of Victoria for three terms in the 1890s. He was implicated in the Texada scandal, was involved in financial irregularities in the construction of the Esquimalt Graving Dock, and in his second term as mayor, was accused of overspending on Victoria's new electric railway. He played a role in the city's smallpox epidemic of 1892 and demanded that Ottawa deal with the approaching cholera epidemic, which was making its way across America. Victoria newspapers alerted Beaven's public to the new contagion:

THE CHOLERA

Its unquestioned existence in and about the Suburbs of Paris. Great Britain fully alive to the dangers. Precautions now being taken. . . . Cholera is making steady headway in Russia, and even the incomplete official returns received, admit that 350 deaths are caused daily by the disease."[1]

Beaven had doubts about the Albert Head Quarantine Station's effectiveness right from the beginning, so he had built a smallpox isolation unit on the site of the Royal Jubilee Hospital. Asked by a reporter what civic officials were doing to stave off this new contagion, he replied:

Of course I am not the Board of Health or the City Council either but I am doing my best to have the city put in good shape. I have, day after day for the past three weeks, urged upon the sanitary officer to see that every place in the city is cleaned up . . . This morning I met with representatives of six companies and have their assurance that Chinatown will be well disinfected . . . There is time enough to make a scare about the cholera when it breaks out here, if it should unfortunately come, but if the Dominion authorities will do their duty, there need be no cholera.[2]

The name *cholera* is derived from the Greek word for bile or anger. Originally, it was the term for one of the four humours identified by Greek physiologists, but it morphed into the name of a bilious form of diarrhea. The epithet Asian Cholera stuck because it began in the Ganges Delta before spreading west along the trade routes through the Caucasus. By 1892, it had claimed 300,000 lives in Russia alone.[3] It soon spread to Spain, France, England, and finally to North America. Cholera appeared in New York in mid-1892 when the ship *Bohemia* docked in the East River and reported fifty-three cases on board. So virulent was the disease that the deadly microbes were still being described at the turn of the twentieth century as, "those puny but terrible little murderers from the Orient."[4]

The result of drinking contaminated water, *Vibrato cholera* caused violent retching and unstoppable diarrhea described as "rice water stools." With the loss of critical amounts of fluid, victims collapsed from radical dehydration. To alleviate the pain from ensuing cramps, they drew themselves into a ball: "With the chin held up against the knees, the victim shrinks into a wizened caricature within a few hours. Soon, ruptured capillaries discolor the skin, turning it black and blue."[5] Physicians reported hearing a soft, whistling sound as breath was drawn between the teeth of comatose patients. Death occurred from shock due to kidney failure and circulatory collapse. Because the final fetal position was unalterable, the body was often buried in this curled-up manner.

Florence Nightingale worked as a volunteer in London during the 1853 epidemic of cholera and believed that infusions of arsenic, mercury, opiates, and bleeding only brought on death more quickly. Other remedies, including vinegar, camphor, horseradish, mint, mustard plasters, leeches, laudanum, and hot baths also proved useless. Nothing worked, least of all quarantine. It would take William Brooke O'Shaughnessy's treatment of radical re-hydration through the injection of a saline solution to bring the disease to its knees.

Ottawa was unable to duck Beaven's imperative and sent health officers on the west coast a flurry of "arrangements." The *Colonist* reported, "Dr. MacNaughton-Jones has received instructions to enforce the regulations to the letter. They apply in exactly the same way to the Albert Head Quarantine Station as to the Grosse Isle station."[6] The dispatches were little more than the usual rhetoric, and Ottawa bureaucrats knew it.

Dr. MacNaughton-Jones had already told the federal government that a whole new quarantine facility was required to quell growing public frustration. Ottawa realized this, but the procurement of a new site was not easy. A location at the southernmost end of Vancouver Island adjacent to the Juan de Fuca Strait was essential. The best place was the William Head Peninsula, but it was not Crown land; it was privately owned and its owner was not going to give it up without a fight.

• • •

THEY DIDN'T CALL ROBERT DE VERE WEIR the "laird" of his estate at William Head entirely without reason. True, he was Scottish, but he was definitely not a nobleman. Robert Weir had left one of the many Highland crofts after the economic collapse during the last phases of the Highland clearances. His ancestors had been forcibly expelled from their ancient glens and settled in Glasgow, Edinburgh, and Dundee. Some capitulated completely and moved to Newcastle and Liverpool. The best move was to immigrate to Canada or Australia.

In 1852, Robert Weir, a widower with six children, moved to Vancouver Island to become a land steward at Craigflower Farm in Victoria. He began to purchase sections of land in Metchosin from Witty's Lagoon to Rocky Point, including the William Head Peninsula. By the 1880s, Robert Weir had bought most of the land around Parry Bay. At last, he felt safe from another eviction and became a Scottish "laird" in his adopted country.

Robert Weir was eighty-four when Ottawa wanted to purchase part of his land for the new station on the William Head Peninsula, so his son John took up the battle. In early 1893, Joseph A. Ouimet, federal minister of public works, offered John $3,000 for sixty acres at the end of the peninsula. John knew it was worth more, so he rejected the offer and went to court. The federal government was not in any mood to dicker, and the file was passed on to Federal Justice Minister John Thompson, soon to be the new prime minister of Canada. Thompson acted quickly, expropriating a larger parcel of land than originally intended, and on March 23, 1893, the William Head Peninsula became the official site of the new quarantine station. John Weir challenged the expropriation in the higher Exchequer Court, but he lost again. A month later, "Messrs Bishop, Sherbourne, and MacFarlane of Victoria secured contracts for the new quarantine buildings and on May 1, work began."[7]

William Head is the southernmost headland of Parry Bay, jutting out into the eastern end of the Juan de Fuca Strait. Southward is Pedder Bay, and barely one kilometre southeast lie the infamous Race Rocks. William Head is far more spectacular than Albert Head, its counterpart at the northern end of Parry Bay, and rises to twenty metres above sea level. Not heavily wooded, the top of the headland is an open plateau with small groves of Douglas fir, Garry oak, and arbutus framing breathtaking views across the strait to the mountains of Washington's Olympic Peninsula. Around its shoreline are finely gravelled beaches, completely shut off from each other by interceding gullies and high cliffs.

The new William Head Quarantine Station would be a far cry from the unworkable facility blundering along at Albert Head. Ottawa had promised that the new site was to be the last word in quarantine control around the world. It boasted that, "in accordance with new sanitary requirements, the centrepiece of the new station was to be a two-story hospital with various 'suspect' detention and isolation quarters located nearby."[8] They would be built, as at Grosse Île, "after the modern style of hospital architecture, with a two-story administration building in the centre, with isolated wings divided by a hallway from the main building."[9] The second floor would have "accommodation for a doctor, caretaker, matron and nurses, with a dispensary, large dining-room and separate sitting room and a large kitchen with proper sculleries, and pantries."[10] Each wing would "be divided into two wards of 15 to 20 beds capacity, each excellently lighted and ventilated. Off each of these wards there was a bathroom and washroom, and here, as in fact throughout the whole building, there was hot and cold running water."[11] The hospital was to be approximately 150 feet long and 90 feet wide, the largest building on-site.

The *Colonist* reported, "Between 300 and 400 metres west of the hospital was the first-class detention building."[12] It housed those first-class shipboard passengers who were well but who might be carriers of deadly contagion. This building was to be by far the most luxurious on the whole site, and the *Colonist* described it as:

> Having long verandas in front with deep overhanging roofs, the main
> door opened into a large dining room, which was to be fitted with
> small tables, the same as the [first-class] dining saloon of a vessel.
> The dining-room took up the whole middle of the building, except the
> rear, which was reserved for the kitchens and pantry appointments.

> Wide hallways, running in both directions from the dinning-room
> led to the bedrooms in sufficient numbers to accommodate without
> crowding 84 people, and in design very like the first-class cabins on a
> ship, except for a fine, large window in each.[13]

The rooms were furnished and fitted with four bunks and would be, according to the plan, very comfortable. Each room had hot and cold water that flowed into mounted porcelain wash basins, providing "guests" with both convenience and privacy in keeping with their special status on board the best of the new trans-Pacific ocean liners. At the end of the hallways were washrooms with flushable lavatories. The whole first-class detention building was heated with two large open fireplaces with smaller, iron wood stoves strategically placed where necessary. In keeping with the strict class system of the day, the first-class detention building would attempt to reflect the shipboard comfort to which the financially and socially privileged classes had become accustomed.

The construction and operation of the Japanese and Chinese detention houses was a very different story. They were "as far removed from the hospital as the European quarters,"[14] and located at the very seaward end of the peninsula. The original plan called for each building to contain its own kitchens, bathrooms, and other conveniences "arranged to combine cleanliness with comfort."[15] What was actually built was cramped dormitory accommodation holding up to three hundred "suspects" in the Japanese building and up to eight hundred detainees in the Chinese quarters. Moreover, in spite of their historical animosities toward each other, the Japanese and Chinese were expected to cook and wash in common open-walled shelters. Confined "Orientals" would be forbidden to mingle with European "guests," so a six-foot-high fence was drawn into the plan to separate the "Oriental" containment houses from the first- and second-class accommodations.

The residence of the chief medical officer, who was now expected to live on the station, was, according to the *Colonist*, a "two-story building well laid out, with five rooms upstairs, large dining-room, drawing room, office, kitchen, etc., and below all, a first-class brick-and-stone cellar. There were spacious verandas on three sides of the house, and with views over the strait to the lights of Port Angeles. The home and cultivated grounds would be delightful with an environment of rare beauty such as are to be seen in a few localities."[16]

Isolated at the end of a small jut of land into Parker Bay was the bacteriological laboratory, with a world-class isolation hospital nearby. Administrative and medical buildings would be built near the proposed main gate. There would be a guardhouse, staff residences, a laundry, a steam plant, a generating station, a pest house or steerage isolation hospital, service sheds, stables, vegetable gardens, and a cemetery. Water was piped in through a four-inch main from a dammed lake three kilometres west of Mary Hill. The water was led first to a 22,000-gallon-capacity water tank that acted as a backup supply in case of fire or line breakage. Terracotta sewer lines ran from each building and connected with cast iron pipes at the water's edge, which ran out to the sea below the low-tide mark. Around the whole 106-acre facility was a ten-foot-high fence with clear and appropriate signage.

The real saving grace of the new William Head Quarantine Station was its permanent wharf. Never again would quarantine officers risk life and limb unloading sick and suspected carriers into small boats during a winter gale. Nor would they have to muscle their way through a crowded dock in Victoria overrun with passengers from other coastal steamers, some of whom might already be carrying infectious diseases. Indeed, the superintendent of construction, William Lorimer, called the wharf "the finest wooden structure of its kind on the coast."[17] With a mean draft of forty-two feet, the five-hundred-foot wharf was sufficient to handle the largest of CPR's new *Empress* fleet, such as the sleek, 450-foot *Empress of India*, which began its trans-Pacific service in 1891. The wharf's eighty-foot wooden pilings were covered in a total of twenty thousand sheets of copper for protection against shipworms before being driven down to bedrock. The wharf was double-braced along its seaward side to protect it against sudden impact.

Along its top ran a small handcart railway, which carried passengers' clothing, baggage, and other effects to the disinfection house nearby. Substantially built with concrete walls and cement floors, the disinfecting chamber inside was built in Victoria by Albion Iron Works and based on a similar facility at the Grosse Île Station. Items to be disinfected were wheeled into the steel chamber, its huge iron doors were sealed, and steam generated in an ante building with a 50-horsepower pump was applied. The local paper asserted, "No germ or microbe survived this experience, and when baggage or anything else came out, it was safe to go anywhere."[18]

Without a wharf, the old Albert Head Quarantine Station finally obtained an inspection tender, the *Earle*, with a portable sulphur-dioxide blast machine on board to fumigate ships at sea, but it arrived too late to be of much use during the smallpox epidemic of 1892. Besides, with its long attached hoses, it was unwieldy and dangerous to use from a small vessel in a seaway. At William Head, the dioxide blast apparatus was transferred to a special hut on the station's wharf. Two smaller jetties provided dock space for two new inspection vessels. Later, it would have a school for the children of station employees.

When the new facility was completed, Dr. MacNaughton-Jones stated, "We now have got what we should have had long ago, and inside of a year, if the Government gives me a free hand, as they have done in the past, we will have a model quarantine station at William Head."[19]

It did not come cheap. The new William Head Quarantine Station cost the federal government $29,539.10, more than twice the amount of the first station at Albert Head. Journalists and citizens alike were only too aware of the horrific consequences that had grown out of the former underfunded facility, and they continually voiced their concerns even as new ground for William Head was being turned. On May 27, 1893, the *Colonist* reported, "It is not to be expected that the arrangements of the William Head Quarantine Station will be on the same scale as those at Grosse Ile, but if quarantine on this side of the continent is to be effective, they must be of the same kind."[20]

Dr. MacNaughton-Jones received the keys to William Head in late August of 1893. He wrote to Ottawa:

The new buildings at William Head were completed about three weeks ago; they still, however, require furnishing, and like all large wooden buildings, have yet some considerable requirements. When these are completed and the furniture in, the quarantine station will be very complete and perfect. The key of my dwelling was handed to me by Mr. Gamble, Chief Engineer of Lands and Works, on the 26th August, and I moved down permanently on the 28th. The three suspect [detention] houses, Caucasian, Chinese, and Japanese, are capable of containing nearly 1,000 people, and the hospital about 80. This contains also several private wards. The water supply is abundant and very perfect. The disinfecting chamber is very good. I would strongly recommend that a telephone be put in the station from town, and the road continued, from the main road to Victoria, to the hospital grounds . . . It is desirable that the furnishings of the buildings be completed as soon as possible; we may have illness at any time.[21]

Dr. MacNaughton-Jones worked hard for the quarantine service during his tenure as chief medical officer, and he was instrumental in restoring good relations between Victoria and its surrounding communities. He tightened the enforcement of existing quarantine regulations, demanded increased vigilance from his medical officers, and argued that unless the Albert Head Station was updated, it should be closed. He was respected and well liked in Victoria, befriending such notables as Judge Matthew Begbie and Henry Crease. In 1894, he averted an epidemic of bubonic plague when he demanded that all ships from Hong Kong, regardless of health certification, be directed to the William Head Station to have all luggage disinfected. He saw to it that all surgeons on Canadian Pacific steamships carried out required vaccinations at their point of departure and began having the baggage from *all* ships from Canton, "the dirtiest city in China," fumigated. Most important of all, he challenged old notions of smallpox quarantine, arguing, "The period of incubation for smallpox varies from five to twenty-six days. I have had cases, myself, of between five and twenty-three days. Consequently, there is no more charm in the reputed fourteen days, than there was in the old days of quarantine."[22]

In a period of fourteen months, Dr. MacNaughton-Jones had given 2,381 ships clearance to enter British Columbia disease free.[23] But he was tired, overworked, and unwell. Despite Ottawa offering him a less taxing position as superintendent of quarantine for British Columbia, he chose to remain working at William Head. He died of a stroke at his home on the station on May 3, 1896, at the age of sixty-four. The city was disconsolate, and "ships anchored in Victoria harbour lowered their flags to half-mast in honour of a physician who had contributed much to safe-guarding the health of his [adopted] country."[24]

His successor, Dr. George Duncan, lasted less than two years. He was appointed as acting superintendent in November 1894, but he made the mistake of neglecting his Dominion superiors at the critical time when Ottawa's involvement needed to be most visible. The *Colonist* reported the outcome on Wednesday, October 14, 1896:

> Dr. Duncan, quarantine officer at William Head has been dismissed. The order-in-council appointing him, passed by the late government, has been cancelled.
>
> Duncan allowed a [quarantined] suspect and a man in charge to come out of quarantine and vote for Earle and Prior in Victoria at the last general election.[25]

Ottawa would not stand for further public scrutiny of any perceived laxity in its west coast quarantine facility. Dr. Duncan had gone on a junket to China without letting his Ottawa superiors know. He was negotiating a policy with Chinese quarantine officials whereby all baggage from that country was to be disinfected while ships were still in Chinese ports. He *had* told his immediate superiors in Victoria of his plans and felt that was enough. But Ottawa either took Duncan's omission as a rebuff or, as the *Colonist* suggested, they dismissed him because at the time the federal government was transitioning from Conservative leadership to Liberal. Duncan was a Conservative, and, as the *Colonist* speculated, Ottawa needed "to make a place for Dr. Watt who was an active Liberal."[26]

Though he was popular in Victoria, Dr. Duncan's explanations didn't wash. Of the charge that he let a man out of quarantine to vote, Dr. Duncan stated that the gentleman was a guard at the station, had been vaccinated, posed no risk, and was free to go. Regardless, Duncan was sacked. It would not be the last time that political patronage raised its head in the service of quarantine.

Dr. Alfred T. Watt was a shoe-in for the vacancy left by Duncan's dismissal. He took charge of the William Head Quarantine Station in late 1897, and within three years of his appointment, the facility's reputation soared. Dr. Watt paid particular attention to the well-being of his patients, and it paid off. The headline said it all: Happiness at William Head.[27]

Roy W. Brown was a reporter with the *Vancouver World*. In September 1900, he was a passenger on the steamer *Walla Walla* when it was quarantined at William Head inbound from San Francisco. With a nose for a good story, Brown did not waste his time while in detention. Here, he felt, was a golden opportunity to pull out all the stops and use his experience to reveal the dirt—the daily operations of life at a quarantine station. It would assure his future reputation as an investigative journalist. What Brown uncovered was a contented society of temporary detainees, "citizens" of William Head who participated fully in daily activities, making their brief stay at the station thoroughly enjoyable. Brown observed that the "inmates" were devoted to Dr. Watt, his abundance of goodwill, his compassion, and his capacity for innovation. There was no "dirt" to be had at William Head.

Brown's dispatches to the *Vancouver Daily World* and the *Colonist* did more than secure Watt's reputation; they stood as a timely commentary upon how life in quarantine had progressed since the days of Albert Head. Brown presented a view of life at William Head that did not whitewash its shortcomings, but rather celebrated the fact that under Dr. Watt's watch, British Columbians could feel safe from the onslaught of infectious disease.

Medical care at the station hospital became the bellwether. "The one smallpox patient is progressing favorably and no more cases have broken out," Brown wrote. Yet he had noticed that different groups of detainees from the *Walla Walla* had departed at different times and was curious. Dr. Watt explained that it was due to different quarantine regulations in effect in Canada and the United States. American regulations allowed for passengers to return to their home country after two weeks of quarantine. Those destined for points in Canada were subject to stricter quarantine laws and required to spend seven more days in detention.

The good cheer was due to Dr. Watt's implementation of a full roster of recreational activities for the suspected carriers of infection who were temporarily confined in quarantine. He selected several events, knowing that camaraderie and exercise were as much a part of good health as was good medicine. One station-organized activity was a weekly baseball game. "The turnout of the residents of the quarantine station at the baseball game yesterday afternoon must have been a record breaker. It was a match between the crew of the *Walla Walla* on one side, and a team picked from her suspected contagious passengers on the other."[28] The "suspect" team was aptly called the "Microbes" and they won handily. "Even excepting the ball game," Brown wrote, "yesterday was an eventful day. The morning was celebrated by the opening of the laundry, away down near the wharf, and half a dozen ladies laboured there industriously all forenoon. The only equipment yesterday was soap and water, but today starch and irons have been obtained, and collars and shirt-fronts are to be homeopathically treated."[29]

When the station's launch arrived back from Victoria with its weekly provisions, Brown noted that Dr. Watt had forgotten nothing:

There were supplies galore; everything from fresh milk to brooms and croquet sets and footballs. At 11 o'clock the launch came from Victoria for the mail. Half the islanders [Brown thought the William Head Peninsula was an island] missed the mail-boat. In quarantine you always tear up your letters if you happen to miss that day's boat. We are not so dreadfully busy but that we can write the same letter over again and add a little more to it. The first adequate supply of stationary also came today, and altogether, conditions were materially improved.

When the Walla Walla, fumigated to her masthead and smelling of sulphur, departed in the hands of a new crew, just afterwards the City of Nanaimo came down from Victoria with a band excursion on board and serenaded us. To a person, we sang "We don't care if you ever come back," and when they called for three cheers for the smallpox suspects, we for a single moment, wished ourselves again in civilization. It was only for a moment, however, for when we remembered where

*we were, we felt sorry for the people who are overpowered with the
questionable liberty of doing what they please.*

    *We are growing happier and more agreeable to one another every
day. As a special kind of Sunday privilege, the gentlemen were yesterday
allowed to visit the nunnery at the opposite side of the island. Sunday
was, by the way, a much easier day to pass than anyone expected. It
rained after breakfast and excursions were, for a time, abandoned.
By the time people in civilization were going to church, however, the
crowd was out in fair weather, exploring the more distant outlooks.*[30]

    Brown noted wryly that those detained passengers who had called
themselves "suspects" had given tongue-in-cheek names to all the outstand-
ing geographic features on the grounds at William Head. One particular
high point with a view of Esquimalt Basin to Victoria's Duntze Head and
Trial Island was named "Hungry Hill." A slight depression in the top of
the headland, protected from summer winds, was named "Dublin Gulch,"
while "Seldom Seen," a great place for reading and contemplation, was a
wooded hollow not far from Dr. Watt's residence.

    Brown soon made friends with one particular fellow traveller, a detained
"suspect," called Dreyfus. He was the cousin of the famous Alfred Dreyfus,
who was accused of giving defence secrets to the Germans in 1894 and
imprisoned on Devil's Island off French Guiana. When the weather was
fair, Dr. Watt allowed William Head's own Dreyfus to pitch a small tent
on a rocky outcropping he called "Devil's Island," yards offshore from the
end of the William Head peninsula. Brown, Dreyfus, and Dr. Watt got on
famously.

    Brown reported to his eager mainland readers that the "inmates" at the
William Head Quarantine Station had created an "Escape Club" with a
mandate of "one victim a day, something on the lines of Stevenson's Suicide
Club."[31] The Escape Club was little more than an intellectual exercise con-
cocted to keep the guards fit. All knew, only too well, that a real escape
violated the true purpose of quarantine—that is, all except one.

    His name was George Récord and he was a German who had recently
worked on the Nicaragua Canal. Brown reported him as saying one evening

in the dining hall, "Whenever I am deprived of my liberty, I always feel like a fool."[32] That first week, other detainees, seeing the utilitarian aspect of the place, had agreed with him. Récord talked continually of leaving from the very first moment he was quarantined and often bragged that he could be away and in Seattle within forty-eight hours. Few took him seriously.

Récord *did* disappear. He made his break on the same evening that the disinfection of all the detainees' personal belongings was to begin. Some wished him well, though most believed he was committing an egregious act. They all knew that temporary quarantine was a major defence against the greater threat of recurring pandemic. Besides, they accepted that life at the station under Dr. Watt's care was most agreeable. Brown wrote, "He, Récord, does not know what he missed. No one would ever think of leaving here unless the business pressure, elsewhere, were enormous."[33] He added, after the episode, "everyone went to the Ladies Hall and there, we were successfully occupied for the remainder of the day."[34] The gentlemen had an eye for the ladies, and Dr. Watt had capitalized upon a safe new means of entertainment.

• • •

THERE WAS A TSUNAMI of immigration to North America from Britain, Europe, and Asia during the early years of the twentieth century. Thousands arrived regularly in sleek, new ocean liners on Canada's west coast. In consequence, the quarantine station at William Head detained more and more suspected carriers who were believed to have associated with fellow travellers sickened by infectious disease. As the detention buildings suffered the inevitable overcrowding, especially those holding steerage passengers, detainees spilled over from dormitories and were housed in tents. As troubling and onerous as such a move could be, several young gentlemen feeling the urge to embrace the new Canadian wilderness actually paid a little extra for the experience of sleeping in a real tent on the edge of nowhere.

In February 1902, one first-class toff who was among the campers added a more sensitive dimension. He told a *Daily Colonist* reporter, "In the summertime, tent life is a recreation not to be despised and quarantined people who care to go to the expense, can be as comfortable as they wished . . . but in the winter it is impossible."[35] For those without means who voyaged toward William Head Station in steerage, it was a situation without choice.

Several well-heeled travellers whose first-class detention quarters were unadorned but quite liveable noticed Dr. Watt's compassion toward those forced to live outside. Some first-class detainees put their considerable reputations on the line by writing letters to Ottawa on Dr. Watt's behalf. One wrote, "Dr. Watt and his devoted services ought to be recognized by placing at his command all the appliances which are necessary to make the enforced detention under his care as little onerous as possible to those unfortunate to have to undergo it."[36] No one during Brown's stay questioned Watt's Herculean efforts to give his temporary guests a positive quarantine experience. For many, the William Head Quarantine Station under Watt's tenure actually provided an opportunity for spiritual restoration as well as a means for discovering new relationships. Along the way, it resulted in a renewed confidence in Canada's newest public health facility.

Dr. Watt also worked to establish a connection with the social elite of Victoria society, and in this context he was not above doing a little diplomatic dancing. The wonder of electricity was all the rage at the time, and with street lighting beginning to show up in many parts of the city, Dr. Watt embraced the technological progress of the new century. In May 1903, on the occasion of the installation of the new electric lighting system for much of the station, Alfred Watt and his wife, Madge, threw a grand ball. The all-night affair made the morning papers.

> The quarantine station at William Head was the scene of an enjoyable ball on Thursday evening when about eighty couples, a large number from the city, were the guests of Dr. and Mrs. A.T. Watt and the quarantine officials. The steamer Earle took those down from the city and returning, landing the merry dancers home about 5:00 am.[37]

During these early years, there was very little real criticism against William Head. Most in Victoria realized the quarantine station existed only because of a continued outpouring of energy and effort directed toward indifferent and often intractable federal officials. Nobody in British

Columbia wanted this hard-won second attempt at a permanent west coast quarantine facility to fail. For many, William Head had become an edifice of pride and sophistication, an emblem of all that was new in public health in Canada, and a symbol of British Columbia's growing modernity. The *Daily Colonist* declared: "William Head is on the route of one of the world's greatest highways, something of which Canada should, under no circumstances, have call to be ashamed."[38]

But the shame would soon come again, and it would come in spades. It would shake Victoria to its foundations and take the cherished leader of a promising new stronghold to an early and enigmatic finish.

CHAPTER 6 // "I'M SORRY, BUT YOU ARE QUARANTINED."

When unhappy Freddie declared himself ready,
to brave all the horrors of strict quarantine.
But little he thought of how dearly he bought,
the circlet alluring of laurel wreath green.

His hard lot repining, his health fast declining,
he wails for his home by the sea.
And curses the lot who first fixed the plot
that doomed him to hunger and full misery.

—"A Quarantine Lament," in *The Daily Colonist*, July 26, 1892

It was inconceivable that Mrs. Richard Cadbury, widow of the famous British chocolate magnate, would succumb to such an uninspired accident. Yet it is equally telling that neither she nor any other passenger of note on the *Empress of India* that day could have escaped what the Grim Reaper wrought at his appointed hour. At least Mrs. Cadbury's four spinster daughters were with her. They were on the last leg of a world tour that had included Africa, India, China, and Japan. They had boarded the *Empress of India* in Yokohama. As dowager champion for the philanthropic arm of the Cadbury chocolate company, the kindly and aging Lady Emma now looked forward to Canada and then home. But when a heavy gale battered the ship in the middle of the Pacific just before dinner on May 21, 1907, Lady Emma fell down the grand staircase. Unconscious, she was carried into the saloon, where she died a few hours later of a brain hemorrhage due to a fractured skull. Her body was embalmed and carried to Vancouver for shipment to England.

Lady Emma's unforeseen death gave rise to fresh, equally inauspicious stirrings among the notables gathered in mourning in the grand saloon. Rumour had reached Scottish physician Sir Alexander Simpson that infectious disease might be onboard. Albert Brassey, head of an aristocratic British family, became nervous, as did John Sellars and Arnold Wilson, managers of the Shanghai and Hong Kong Dock companies. The Bell-Irvings from Vancouver, their governess, and a number of retiring diplomats, missionaries, and military officers all shared the growing unease. The *Colonist* noted, "As the *Empress of India* steamed for the Strait of Juan de Fuca, there was fear among a large complement of passengers that the liner might be quarantined."[1] Their concern was not unfounded.

The Reverend Emerson knew death only too well. For much of his adult life he had been a missionary in China, and had encountered poverty where children especially succumbed to the diseases of malnutrition. He was returning to England with his wife and two young infants, and had alerted the ship's surgeon some days before that his children were listless and had a persistent fever.

The quarantine station at William Head was incomplete in 1907, though its hospitals, detention facilities, fumigation units, and bathhouses were in place and equipped to handle most inbound epidemics. Three days later, as the ship steamed toward the light at Cape Flattery, provisions for the *Empress*'s arrival were well underway. The telegrapher in the wireless office on board had already contacted the lighthouse at Race Rocks, and Captain O.P. Marshall understood the keeper's reply. It was not necessary yet to fly the yellow flag of quarantine on the foremast, or place a red lantern over a white lamp above the flag until medical officers had joined the ship. Lightkeeper W.P. Daykin had telephoned William Head with news of the reported sickness directly. Sooner than estimated, the *Empress of India* arrived off William Head just after dawn on May 27, 1907.

• • •

DR. WATT, THE STATION'S chief medical officer for ten years, was alert yet comfortable. In 1900, he had instituted a policy of meeting all inbound ships with quarantine officers in the station's tender as they slowed off Parry Bay. That way, all "Orientals" and other passengers were examined *before* a ship needed to be sent to the quarantine wharf. If a vessel was found to be contagion free, it was cleared where it was and could carry on almost without stopping. Shipping companies and local businesses alike appreciated his new time-saving procedure, but it was dangerous. Even in daylight and fair weather, the rolling swells of Juan de Fuca Strait made any boarding risky. In darkness and foul weather, it could be downright deadly.

William Head's initial quarantine boat was the *Earle*, a steam-powered tug just over forty feet long with a small wheelhouse, galley, and berths for three. But it was not suitable for the open strait, and there were many times during the winter gales when the skipper dared not leave the dock. "The *Earle* was not the right class of steamer for boarding vessels out in the open with a high sea running," Dr. Watt wrote.[2] By 1903, the *Earle* had worn out its engine, so William Head acquired another tender, *Madge*. The *Madge* was similar to the *Earle,* but more reliable and powerful. Yet even it rolled uneasily in a seaway.

Just beyond Race Rocks, an inbound ship requiring quarantine clearance reduced speed and slung out over its side a huge metal gangway, a set of steel stairs angled in such a manner that the small boarding platform at its base was level with the seas. As the tender manoeuvred alongside the great ship, quarantine officers watched for the right moment to step onto the swaying platform. With medical bags in hand, they didn't waste any time reaching a ship's main deck.

In good weather the waves were smaller, but there were still perils that awaited those in the quarantine service who ventured out into the seas in small boats. Deadheads were products of the booming west coast forest industry, single logs that broke free from their log booms while being towed across the numerous exposed inlets of Puget Sound and the Gulf Islands. Lost in the tidal currents that swept around Vancouver Island, they soon become waterlogged, partially submerged, and invisible. In foul weather, rough seas caused them to rise and fall in the waves so they were a little more conspicuous, but in calm seas, these saturated, Parthenon-sized, old-growth obelisks of fir and cedar sank vertically just beneath the surface, ready to strike any vessel on their bearing. Like a torpedo, a deadhead could burst a hole through a small hull, causing it to founder it in minutes. If the heaving seas slowly laid a deadhead on its side, it could just as easily roll underneath a hull and sever a boat's rudder and propeller in seconds.

Scrambling up the towering side of an ocean liner or freighter during a full winter gale was another matter completely. Here, the gangway staircase was useless in that it would have been smashed to pieces by a ship's hull in the constant rolling. In heavy weather, the gangway was replaced by a Jacob's ladder, or pilot's ladder, which hung like a huge net when unrolled from the main deck down the hull to the water. A Jacob's ladder resembled a rope ladder, except that it had wooden rungs interspaced with longer and wider boards to prevent it from twisting. The boards also held it far enough off a ship's side in order for a boarder to gain a proper foothold. As the quarantine tender approached, quarantine officers moved on deck and stood by the lifelines. Wearing ungainly foul-weather gear and kapok life preservers, they waited until the boat rose to the top of a particularly large wave, grasped a rope rung high above the foam, and scrambled up for dear life. In the same instant, the tender powered astern so as not to crush the hapless officials as it rose again on the next wave. Alone above the seething brine, the medical officers warily made their way up the boarding ladder and over the rail to the safety of a ship's deck.

• • •

IN THE PRE-DAWN DARKNESS of May 27, 1907, the seas were calm as Dr. Watt boarded the *Empress of India* in the strait. He confirmed that the two children in question did have an infectious disease, but their temperatures and the size of their rashes made him believe they had chickenpox and not smallpox. Mrs. Emerson was beside herself, but she was calmed by Dr. Watt's easy manner and optimistic prognosis. Dr. Watt informed them that, nonetheless, the family would have to be quarantined.

More serious was Watt's examination of two Japanese steerage passengers who were seriously ill. Both were in pain, could hardly walk, seemed confused, and had some tingling in their hands and feet. In one, Dr. Watt thought he noticed an irregular heartbeat. Unsure of a diagnosis until more tests could be done, he decided that they, too, would need to be detained. The ship was ordered to the station's wharf.

Some passengers, when they learned of the situation, began to recall recent associations, especially the Bell-Irvings' young governess. She had had afternoon tea with Mrs. Emerson, and wondered if she might have caught the children's sickness. Mrs. Wilson had also met the Reverend Emerson, and tried to remember if she had shaken his hand one morning after chapel. Dr. Watt would speak to them all. In total, 15 first-class passengers, 7 second-class tourist passengers, and 130 Chinese passengers who had travelled in enclosed third class (one step above open steerage) would also be landed and confined. Beyond the passengers' detainment, their clothing and cabined baggage would also need to be unloaded and disinfected. It was uncertain if the ship would require fumigation before being allowed to proceed.

Meanwhile, back at the William Head Quarantine Station, it was 5:45 a.m. and final preparations for landing the *Empress of India* were underway. Thick fog hung in the strait as Mr. Poole, station superintendent, pulled the main breaker to illuminate the station's four-hundred-foot wharf. The street lamps leading to the dormitories for detained steerage passengers were not yet fully electrified, so they had to be lit by hand. Fires under the boilers in the steam plant were ordered begun and stoked. Other workers unlocked a smaller shed near the wharf and began to prepare powerful disinfectant chemicals, such as chlorine and sulphur, used in the disinfection and fumigation processes. It was important to get the proportions of the disinfectant solution exactly right as it would be pumped to the bathhouse near the end of the pier. Then towels, slippers, and bathrobes for first-class passengers needed to be counted and readied.

By 1907, ships were cleared through William Head twenty-four hours a day. Consequently, the station had two full-time physicians on duty to share the load. With such a large number facing detention this particular morning, Dr. Alexander, along with customs officer McMinn, would meet Dr. Watt and the *Empress of India* at the wharf. The full complement of station guards would have been roused from their quarters near the main gate by the superintendent's wife and directed to the pier.

Suddenly, like the soundless raising of the curtain on *Madame Butterfly*, the glistening presence of the *Empress of India* ghosted silently through the early morning fog to the wharf. With the giant figurehead barely visible above the bow, its lines were slung over the dockside bollards and made fast. On the master's order, the second officer moved the large brass indicator of the chain-driven mechanical telegraph to the "finish with engines" position. Moments later, the second engineer replied, and the repeater indicator rang out, confirming the captain's wish. All was stilled.

Dr. Alexander and Dr. Watt conferred briefly on the bridge. The Emerson children would not immediately be placed in the station's hospital but kept under close observation with their parents in the first-class isolation building. The two steerage passengers would be moved to another isolation pest house, while the rest from steerage would be directed to the Chinese and Japanese dormitories. Dr. Alexander and Captain Marshall decided that the stewards should assemble the first-class passengers needing to be detained under the canvas-covered promenade deck. Dr. Alexander also mentioned that he would be back to examine the ship's log for the records of its inbound ports of call, the crew vaccination papers, and cargo manifest when he had the chance. Captain Marshall nodded. Dr. Watt confirmed an assembly station for steerage passenger detainees where he would check their vaccination certificates and give further inoculations where necessary. Things were getting done. In a flash, both Dr. Watt and Dr. Alexander were gone.

On the promenade deck, Lord Brassey noticed a line of Chinese passengers being led off the ship in single file into the drizzle and morning darkness. Each drooped as they carried something very large and flat on their backs, which made them appear like a line of dark beetles.

Those first- and second-class passengers who had no contact whatsoever with the Emersons were, in this instance, allowed to remain on board the *Empress of India* at the wharf. Normally, Dr. Watt would have insisted that every person on board—officers, crew, and passengers of every class—be landed for the duration of the quarantine period. However, he was certain that the children had chickenpox and felt confident that only 15 of the 146 first-class passengers had had any contact with them or their parents. He also decided that of the 602 passengers in steerage, the 472 who travelled in makeshift cabins called *enclosed* steerage posed no threat of being carriers of their disease. Only the 130 Chinese who were in *open* (dormitory) steerage, and hence inevitably mixed with the two Japanese, were landed and detained. Dr. Watt suspected that even their illness may not be contagious, though he had heard of a recent smallpox epidemic in Kobe, Japan, where one hundred new cases were being detected daily. By year's end, Kobe had reported over two thousand cases with a mortality rate of over 50 percent.[3] China and Japan had a poor reputation in combating infectious disease, and Dr. Watt was not taking any chances.

First to receive disinfecting showers were the fifteen first-class passengers. They were taken to a long red-brick building beside the wharf that housed the power plant, changing rooms, and steam-sterilizing retorts. At one end of the building, separated by a partition, was the bathhouse. There, ladies and gentlemen were asked politely to label items such as pocket watches, chains, cravat pins, necklaces, jewellery, coins, and wallets and place them into a small, numbered tray that would be received by an attendant. Then, in separate dressing areas, they were told to remove each piece of clothing, attach to it an identification ticket, and place it in a small nearby metal cart standing on rails at the door. Half-naked, they waited for a shower. The warm sterilizing shower contained a weak solution of bichloride, which made the skin slippery to the touch and burned if it entered the eyes. As stark and as limited as these facilities were, they were a big improvement over the two wooden washtubs that had been used at Albert Head some ten years before.[4]

Upon leaving the shower, detainees were given warm towels and a blanket-like kimono and ushered through yet another partition into a small room to wait for their disinfected clothing. It was important that the two groups of quarantined people—those about to go *into* the showers and those already "cleansed"—did not mix. More critical was that the partitions separating these two parts of the disinfection building be kept sealed and airtight. Cracks and holes in the interior walls were highways for pathogens and could lead to immediate reinfection. The Northern Pacific Steamship Company's vessel *Victoria* had several patients reinfected in this manner in 1896, so Dr. Watt had the whole structure fully lined a year before the *Empress of India* arrived. A separate bathhouse was still under construction.

The disinfection of clothing occurred in the steam-sterilizing unit. Two metal cars sitting on a narrow-gauge railway that ran along the wharf were loaded with clothing and bedding from the ship and wheeled into a large steel retort. With the door sealed, an electric pump withdrew fifteen cubic inches of air from its interior. This negatively pressurized chamber then received blasts of steam, which raised the inside temperature to over 100°C for over two hours. Articles of clothing or valuables that might be damaged by steam were submerged in a bichloride of mercury solution, immersed in naptha, or saturated with the fumes of burning sulphur for at least six hours.

The so-called waiting room had only a few chairs and little else. A wood stove did provide a modicum of heat during the winter months, but even on that foggy May morning, it would have been cold. Here, all were given yet another blanket-kimono and told to place the slippers, towels, and robes they had just used in another empty cart, which would be taken back through the retort and sterilized. Three hours passed before most of the steamed clothing was returned, and no doubt by this time Lord and Lady Brassey, the Emersons, and several others would have felt the sting of cold. Clothes in hand, they followed an attendant up from the wharf along a pathway wet with drizzle to their cabins in the first-class detention building that was to be their home for the next two, or possibly three, weeks.

Along the way, Lord Brassey again witnessed a straggling Chinese man bearing his heavy burden across his back. Suddenly the mystery was solved. The Chinese were carrying their mattresses!

By 1907, the first-class detention house had been subdivided into twenty-eight smaller rooms or "cabins" all under the same roof, and though every attempt had been made to make them comfortable, they were a far cry from the first-class cabins on board a liner as luxurious as the *Empress of India*. Roughly measuring seven by nine feet, each cabin had bare-plank floors with hospital-white wooden walls. Each contained a small cabinet on which sat a single coal-oil lamp, four steel-sprung bunk beds, a chair, and a mirror. The beds had no bedding, there were no pictures, rugs, or other refinements.

In contrast, Lord and Lady Brassey's first-class accommodation on the *Empress of India* had boasted over 150 square feet of luxury. It sported a huge, high bed with captain's drawers underneath, a large walnut wardrobe, a secretary desk and chair, a chesterfield, a smaller late-baroque writing table, and two upholstered matching chairs with cabriole legs. Finely crafted wainscotting covered the lower half of the walls, and an East India rug made the floor soft underfoot. There was a large-bladed electric ceiling fan; electric lights; and a fully opening brass porthole, its wonderfully high view of the passing sea shaded by brocade, ivory-coloured curtains held back by a matching sash. On the wall above the bed was a framed painting of Queen Victoria. On the writing table were two printed cards, the larger one outlined the menu and dress code for the evening meal and the times of the sittings in the first-class dining room. The smaller card contained the name of the Brasseys' personal stewardess, Miss C. Green, who had written "pleased to serve you" at the bottom in immaculate script. Fresh flowers were delivered daily.

The accommodations in the first-class detention building, though far from luxurious, *were* fairly comfortable. Fresh bedding had been brought off the ship and an attendant had lit the fireplace, which was blazing away in the common room at the end of the hall. The room had enough large tables and chairs to seat fifty for meals, but it was also used as a smoking and reading room with two armchairs and bookshelves, which currently stood empty. However, the ship's library was well stocked with books that were made available to the detainees. The first-class detention house at the station was among the first to be electrified some years before, but winter gales often blew down the lines, so two oil lamps stood nearby on a table. The *Daily Colonist* was delivered to the first-class quarters daily and most read it with great amusement. The telephone, which had only just been installed, had not yet been hooked up, so Mrs. Watt generously offered to allow her "guests" the use of the private phone in her own home for "messages of urgency."

There were a few other perks. All the food for the first-class detainees was prepared by chefs on board the *Empress of India*, and delivered to the "guests" in their common room with all the appropriate shipboard condiments. Menus included "Consomme a la Jerusalem, Filets des Canards aux olives, Rise de veau a la Matégon, Yorkshire pudding and Roast Beef, Pudding King George, Apple Hedgehog, and Gelle au vin d'Oporto."[5] In short, there was "everything from smoked oysters to bird's-nest soup."[6] One thing that the first-class detention house did not have was live music to accompany dinner. The ship's orchestra remained on board and played their evening program of a nocturne, a fantasia, and selections from an opera to those privileged enough to have access to the *Empress*'s white-and-gold–trimmed grand saloon and lucky enough not to have been detained ashore.

For those who were detained, there was a full calendar of games and walks about the station, not to mention the daily visits and examinations by Dr. Watt and his staff, who had a reputation for being affable and helpful. If the situation was accepted with civility and forbearance, the experience of quarantine at William Head could be quite pleasant. Some notables, however, chose only to see the worst, and felt their incarceration to be an affront to their class. One group of first-class passengers on the *Empress of China*, quarantined at the station in 1898, complained to the local papers:

> We were taken out of our comfortable cabins in batches of twelve or so at a time; stripped naked and subjected to a foul chemical bath; our clothes taken from us to be fumigated and baked, we were [left] sitting meanwhile in a shed, clad in an old blanket gown and pair of slippers, which had been previously used to cover the naked-ness of, no one knows, how many Chinese.
>
> Neither ladies nor children, no matter how delicate, were to be excepted from this odious and revolting operation.
>
> The Chinese steerage passengers, who are being driven into the bathing shed, where, after being parboiled, they make their appearance on the rocks behind to don the blanket coat. Their appearance is highly picturesque and affords a fine subject for the cameras on board.[7]

Such churlish pique was not uncommon. When it occurred again among first-class passengers in 1913, it would have far more catastrophic consequences.

Chinese and Japanese passengers who travelled steerage class (third-class enclosed or open) on the *Empress of India* did not fare as well. Besides group showers, they faced accommodation on cots in unheated, bare dormitories, each holding more than a hundred people. Where their numbers outstripped the beds, tents accommodated the excess. Confined steerage passengers were fed mostly rice, but it was prepared for them, on this voyage at least, on the *Empress of India* and delivered. Asian passengers who were confined from other ships often had to prepare their own food.

Hong Len Jung travelled to Vancouver on the *Empress of India* in steerage in 1911, and spoke of the exorbitant prices crewmembers charged just for basic nourishment:

> [On board], there was rice . . . not very tasty . . . just all stirred up together in a wok. You were never full because they, the Chinese crew, wanted you to buy it from them. Those sailors sold rice to us with Chinese sausage and salted duck eggs. They never made good food for us for the regular meals. Your regular meal was at 5:00 – 6:00 pm. They, the sailors, would sell their food to us around 10:00 pm at night. That was the good food. The Chinese cooks and sailors saved the food and took it from the ship's stores to sell to us. They charged us 20 cents a bowl.[8]

The Chinese and Japanese dormitories at William Head shared a partially covered common cook shed equipped with several twenty-five-gallon black iron cooking pots. The daily ration of rice was augmented by vegetables, birds, and other small animals sometimes poached from surrounding farms. Such foraging under Dr. Watt's tenure at William Head was uncommon, but it did make a difference. Yet, even with the extra spices and noodles that always seemed to appear, the resulting thin soups, dim sum, and stir-fries never adequately fed the undernourished Asians thousands of miles from their homeland.

In spite of the conditions, most detained Asians accepted their fate with aplomb and enjoyed Dr. Watt's daily visits—repressing their laughter as the good doctor attempted to pronounce simple Cantonese phrases and delighting in his theatrical efforts to communicate in gestures. As often as he could, Dr. Watt brought them eggs, chickens, and geese from his small nearby farm.

• • •

WHEN PASSENGERS WERE DETAINED at William Head, their cabined baggage was disinfected. If deadly contagion was on board, the whole vessel and its cargo was subject to fumigation. Rats, worms, cockroaches, and other vermin all carried deadly microbes, and they all made secret homes on the ships that regularly crossed the equator and international dateline. Tempted aboard along the mooring lines, or covered in the folds and layers of silk, fruit, tea, opium, and other general cargo—which on this particular trip of the *Empress of India* represented over a million dollars—the pests soon inhabited every part of a ship. Some carried pathogens with impunity and infected unsuspecting passengers through a bite, a scratch, or excreta. Others transmitted disease through a short drink of human blood. When deadly contagion was discovered on the *Empress of India*, only the fumes of deadly chemicals could reach the infected vermin hiding in the ship's cracks, crannies, and crevasses; however, fumigation was a complex, time-consuming, and dangerous process.

The gas of burning sulphur dioxide was the operative agent. It was used for fumigating all ships at most quarantine stations prior to the First World War because it was cost-effective and successful, even when carried out by relatively untrained technicians. Sulphur dioxide was the gas of choice at William Head for many years. Sealed wooden casks of caked yellow sulphur were kept under lock and key in a small shed located near the wharf. One pound of sulphur was used for every one thousand cubic feet of space to be fumigated and was then ground into a fine powder. Small ceramic pots were filled with the powder and depressed at the top. These "flowerpots" of sulphur were then placed into larger, shallower wooden containers meant to separate them from cold and often damp metal. Once the pots were strategically placed throughout a ship, each depression was filled with ethyl alcohol, a priming agent used for ignition.

When sulphur is exposed to water, it is extremely corrosive, so direct contact between the chemical and metal-hulled ships, and indeed any metal structure upon which the pots of sulphur were placed, was to be avoided. Set improperly, the fumigant chemical could spill onto a damp metal bulkhead and eventually eat its way through the partition. If sulphur lay directly against the damp steel plate of a ship's hull and was ignored, it could, in time, send a ship to the bottom of the sea.

When larger spaces of a ship such as the cargo holds required fumigation, all the hatches were first sealed and covered with waterproof tarpaulins. Passengers' steamer chests, large suitcases, and other moveable cargo were removed from their storage racks and scattered about. Sometimes, baggage or boxed cargo was opened. Huge sulphur pots filled with a maximum of thirty pounds of sulphur were fitted into wooden receptacles and placed throughout an area where vermin were known to nest. In smaller spaces, such as steerage cubicles, cabins, or lockers, the standard "flowerpot" of sulphur was used. Here, too, the areas needed to be completely airtight, and it was the fumigant technician's job to seal all doors, portholes, and hatchways from the inside with strips of adhesive paper. When all was ready, he lit the ethyl alcohol and made sure it ignited the sulphur. Without dawdling, he let himself out of the one remaining uncovered door and sealed it from the outside.

The fumigation period varied from six to twelve hours, with a further twenty-four hours required for ventilation before mattresses, baggage, and cargo were deemed safe to touch. Representative dead specimens of all vermin and insects were collected, turned over to the station's bacteriologist, examined for known microscopic pathogens, and burned. Even with adequate ventilation, anything connected to the fumigation process would reek of rotten eggs for days.

Canvas bags containing letters and parcels were fumigated separately. The bags, loosened at the top, were placed in special carts and were subject to the same fuming gas. The process would effectively stall the delivery of anything carried by Royal Mail for up to a week.

In 1897, Dr. Watt received approval to construct a larger, 150-foot-square sulphur blast building beside the wharf in which huge amounts of sulphur were burned in a special furnace. The deadly gas was pressurized and pumped in long hoses, man-hauled by technicians in protective clothing, to the necessary locations throughout a ship at the wharf. The building also contained a special "sulphur room" capable of holding the baggage of several hundred people. But this pressurized sulphur process, in its early years at least, often broke down and was considerably more dangerous for technicians than the less effective, but safer "flowerpot" technique.

Dr. Watt also asked for a formic aldehyde generator for William Head, as this particular gas was considered safer and faster than sulphur dioxide, but his request was refused because the active chemical, paradichloroben-zene, required heating to 20°C. The process was expensive and required a thorough drying of all apparel, so it was not popular on the west coast. In 1913, Dr. Walker suggested that carbon monoxide gas wafted about through hoses was better than burning sulphur for the purpose of fumigation. Thankfully, his idea was also rejected.

Toward the end of the First World War, another, more powerful chemical came into use, but it was expensive and even more lethal than sulphur dioxide. A hydrogen cyanide gas compound, which sold under the trade name of Zyklon B, began to be adopted by quarantine stations with sufficient traffic to warrant its expense and risk. Hydrogen cyanide is one of the world's most dangerous fumigants. Indeed, a derivative of it was used in the gas chambers of Auschwitz during the Second World War. The gaseous reaction was in itself similar to that of burning sulphur, but it required much less preparation and was much more potent. A commercially prepared mixture of sodium cyanide and diluted sulphuric acid was sealed within an airtight tin. When the tin was opened, the chemicals immediately reacted with the air, resulting in the production of deadly hydrocyanic acid gas (HCN).

For ships' holds, saloons, and cabins, HCN and sulphuric acid was purchased premixed with diatomaceous earth or ground wood pulp and packed into airtight tins called "bombs." For small areas such as lockers, Zyklon B was supplied as pellets or diskettes packed in similar airtight containers. Specially machinated can openers, unique to the Zyklon B process, fitted only a particular batch of containers and accompanied each shipment. The trained attendant, aware of the instant deadly effect of hydrocyanic acid gas, had to be sure a space was cleared and sealed before opening a "bomb." To kill everything in sight, complete fumigation with HCN required twenty-four hours followed by a ventilation period of ten hours. Zyklon B, however, was very temperature-sensitive, and personnel using it had to wear a full protective suit. Gas masks were required, but they proved to be effective for only ten minutes as the deadly fumes permeated even the finest charcoal-mesh filters. Zyklon B was used at William Head, but not until well after the First World War, and then only during the warmer summer months.

• • •

THOUGH DEATH HAD CERTAINLY stalked this particular Pacific crossing of the *Empress of India,* the Emersons, aristocrats, businessmen, and even those in steerage got away lucky. Lady Emma Cadbury was gone, but the Emerson children and the two Japanese passengers from steerage were spared. The children fully recovered from chickenpox a few days after being quarantined, and all those who had contact with the family remained free of the disease for the duration of their confinement.

Dr. Watt was right; the two Japanese passengers never had a contagious infectious disease. They had developed a vitamin deficiency, likely caused by a diet consisting mainly of polished white rice, which had become mass-produced for the world market in Japan during the last quarter of the nineteenth century. Ordinary "paddy rice" was removed from its husks in huge milling machines, making it readily available and cheaper for almost everyone. But the milling process also "polished" the kernels, removing most of its nutritious value, whereas ordinary, sun-dried paddy rice, parboiled the old way, remained wholesome *and* full of the dietary requirement of vitamin B_1. Polishing white rice simply processed its vitamins away to nothing.

Dr. Watt wouldn't have known this, but he would have known that beriberi had spread among armed forces and prisoners of war in Southeast Asia during the 1890s. They were fed polished white rice as the main staple of their diet. He might have also read about chickens in Indonesia that lost the use of their legs when fed rice milled by the new process. Chickens fed on brown rice remained healthy or recovered completely if they did fall ill.

Microscopic analysis of mucous specimens from the two quarantined Japanese passengers did *not* reveal a bacterial, acid-fast agent, ruling out lepromatous leprosy and other infectious diseases with similar symptoms to those the passengers exhibited. Watt thought about their diet, jobs, and the locale in which they lived in Japan, and diagnosed the pair with beriberi. He fed them up and let them go. All the other Asian steerage passengers had remained healthy, even jovial, during the short period of their confinement and all were ultimately released.

Because of Dr. Watt's diagnosis and the vigilance of his medical officers, the *Empress of India* did not require fumigation on this particular voyage, and it was soon on its way to Vancouver. It would not be the last time that the great ship avoided quarantine at the William Head Station. Even more famous CPR steamships would be halted and subject to the same procedures that awaited Reverend Emerson and those who travelled with him.

CHAPTER 7 // THE STRANGE, SAD CASE OF ALFRED TENNYSON WATT

There is no leprosy but what you speak.

—William Shakespeare, *Timon of Athens*, 4.3

I t is not uncommon for a father to name his first-born son after someone significant—a celebrity, a luminary, someone that might inspire the child. Hugh Watt named his first son after Alfred Lord Tennyson. It would turn out to be a fitting and almost uncanny choice in that the life of Alfred Tennyson Watt, chief medical officer at the William Head Quarantine Station from 1897 to 1913, embodied those same elements of duty and alienation that were the themes of Queen Victoria's favourite poet. More incredible was that Alfred Tennyson Watt possessed Tennyson's conservatism, love of nature, sentimentality, and nervous sensitivity. In Tennyson's case, these qualities generated a lifelong poetic creativity. In Watt's case, these same sensibilities led to a downfall that many believed was caused by a calculated character assassination.

Born on a farm near Meaford in Grey County, Ontario, in 1868, Alfred Tennyson Watt expressed the best qualities of an English aristocrat of the Victorian era. Imbued with a clear sense of noblesse oblige, he was charming, intelligent, taciturn, and tough. At Upper Canada College, he excelled in rugby and played on the all-star varsity team while studying medicine at the University of Toronto. By the time he graduated, he had established a reputation as one of Ontario's top-ten rugby players. While he was a student, his physician father moved to Elko, British Columbia, to farm, practise medicine, and become a long-time Conservative member of the British Columbia legislature. Alfred followed his father west and began a practice in Victoria, initially in partnership with Dr. Milne. He soon joined the Victoria Rugby Club, opened an independent medical office, and shared a place on Fort Street with his good friend, Judge Lampman. He entered the social circle of Victoria's new gentry, but a professional life among the privileged was not enough, so he distanced himself from their excesses and set about pursuing a more personal dream. Like his father, he wanted to raise sheep on a farm in the country. For all his urbane class, Alfred Tennyson Watt preferred a more rustic life.

The nineteenth-century zeitgeist was shaped by two antagonistic forces: a belief in progress and an arresting sense of doubt. The sense of mystery and obedience that opened the century would give way to audacity and entitlement at its close. This century saw the discovery of the source of the Nile and the fabled Timbuktu, and penetration of the looming vastness of the Northwest Passage. It also produced calotype photography, the pneumatic tire, the Plimsoll Line, antiseptics, and that icon of capitalism, the mechanical cash register. The philosophical and political convictions of the period resulted in the suffragette movement, franchise for the working class, and primary education for all. Even Darwin's theories, though troubling for many, were touted by some as a validation of progress. And the British felt it was their "natural" right to assume leadership in a world where the endless sun of empire set only on the prejudice that all things *not* British were primitive and uncivilized.

But there was anxiety: over the alarming migration to cities with their growing abject poverty, over the desecration of the natural landscape —and over God. Even the earnestness of the Baptists, Methodists, Congregationalists, and Nonconformists could not entirely assuage the ontological unease that lay beneath the notion of progress.

As Poet Laureate in this age of progress, Alfred Lord Tennyson celebrated the achievements of his time, but he also wrote of its growing alienation. His wistful, often dispirited voice spoke eloquently of the struggle for faith and understanding in a world full of striving and self-satisfaction.

At twenty-five, Alfred Tennyson Watt reunited with Margaret Robertson. "Madge" and Alfred were students together at the University of Toronto at a time when few women pursued post-secondary education. She was from a well-established Ontario family, the daughter of celebrated Collingwood lawyer Henry Robertson. They married in December 1893, and together they would have a farm, raise two sons, and establish separate notable careers. Madge became a lecturer, writer, and organizer in the New Women's movement and would later win many honours, including an Order of the British Empire. Alfred would become a prominent figure in infectious disease control and raise sheep. Madge Watt was the crusader; Dr. Alfred Tennyson Watt was more private.

Was it his boyhood in rural Ontario that made him self-reliant and taciturn, or was it medicine itself? It's hard to know, but Dr. Watt, though easy among Victoria's high society, paid little heed to the politics of privilege. Those who knew him well described him as egalitarian-minded and soft-spoken. He remained the quintessential yeoman farmer—self-reliant, creative, and strong. He was a man of great perception and pride, and others' exploitation of these traits became his undoing.

It was during the smallpox epidemic of 1892 that Alfred Watt first established himself as a physician of remarkable insight and initiative. As health officer for the City of Victoria, he examined and vaccinated hundreds of passengers from coastal steamers in and out of Victoria. He travelled to Gretna, Manitoba, and diagnosed the missionary, Miss Calder, with smallpox, returning with her to the Albert Head Quarantine Station. A year later, he was appointed secretary to the Provincial Board of Health. There, he revised the province's quarantine regulations and was asked to head the committee to write British Columbia's first Health Act. Those on the committee all conceded that the act was largely the work of Dr. Alfred Tennyson Watt.

During this time, he also revealed his considerable moral fibre. In the fall of 1892, Dr. Watt submitted a detailed invoice for $1,342.50 to Victoria's council for medical services far beyond his job description. City officials tried to weasel out of paying the invoice, declaring the fees "degrading" and of "trade union prices." Begrudgingly, they offered him a lower amount and believed he would eat humble pie. Watt refused to accept the offer, alleging it was full of reactionary malice. He forwarded the account to the attorney general's office, claiming, "no satisfactory reason has been assigned why the original arrangement should not be adhered to."[1] A champion of decency, he would not allow an ideology of pettiness to pass for sound judgment. The bill was paid in full forthwith.

Dr. Watt was a shoe-in for the position of chief medical officer of the William Head Quarantine Station when Dr. Duncan was dismissed in 1897. He bought land nearby for his intended farm and lived permanently at the station. Farming would become his precious avocation, but the William Head Quarantine Station became his passion.

Within five years of his appointment, Alfred Watt had made great strides. In 1901, he established a Christmas fund, supported by shipping companies, for those travellers and their children who had the misfortune to be detained at William Head over the holiday period. A year later, he built new accommodations for the station's full-time guards and constructed a new detention building solely for Chinese steerage passengers. He upgraded the bacteriological laboratory, created a smaller "cottage" hospital especially for smallpox cases, and began negotiations with Ottawa to electrify the whole station. That year, the William Head Quarantine Station inspected 442 vessels inbound for British Columbia, and none cleared the station with infectious diseases still on board. Watt broadened MacNaughton-Jones's plan to have the baggage of steerage passengers fumigated in most Asian ports of departure, visited American quarantine stations in Puget Sound and the American side of Juan de Fuca Strait, and was instrumental in developing the National Quarantine Officers of the Pacific Northwest.[2]

In January 1901, the *City of Seattle* was quarantined at William Head and over three hundred first- and second-class passengers were detained. They were so pleased with Dr. Watt's attention and treatment during their confinement that they petitioned Ottawa to change the regulations forbidding officials from accepting gifts. The Canadian government quickly made a special dispensation and bathed in the afterglow. Dr. Watt and Mr. Wallace, a resident male nurse, received engraved gold watches.[3]

It wasn't all roses, though. In February 1902, the British Columbia Board of Trade received criticism from a group of first-class passengers who had been held at William Head. They claimed that their valuables had gone missing, soiled clothing was simply allowed to accumulate in great heaps on the wet floors of the bathhouse, and the water for their disinfectant showers was freezing. When the complaints hit the newspapers, Dr. Watt used the criticism to educate the general public in the ways of quarantine health.

He asserted in a public letter that bacteria were ubiquitous, so even valuables such as watches and jewellery were removed and fumigated separately. Clothing was purposefully left in heaps, he wrote, simply because if pegs had been provided, the detainees would have forgotten to leave their clothes behind for disinfection. The bathwater cooled because the building housing the steam-heating unit for the whole station was under-insulated and still under construction. Chagrined, all the complainants admitted later that their possessions had been returned. As a gesture of good faith, Dr. Watt publicly offered to buy new suits and sweaters for those inconvenienced. He wryly wrote that "they could afford to write a cheque for more money than the whole station was worth."[4] At this point in his career, Dr. Watt had become sufficiently confident to be a little irascible with those who confused a quarantine station with a Mediterranean resort.

Within ten years of Watt's arrival, the William Head Quarantine Station had been transformed, though its mandate had not changed. For Alfred Tennyson Watt, the preventing of infectious diseases from entering British Columbia and the equitable treatment of all those detained in his care remained supreme. He took advantage of the natural beauty of the William Head Peninsula to create pathways through the scattered copses of red cedars and alders. He placed benches on rocky outcroppings facing the Olympic Mountains and planted an English garden near the hospital. On high, more open spaces he created a playing field for the children of detainees, and in 1909, he opened a school for the children of station staff. For first-class detainees, he even created a golf course. Aesthetics and exercise, he knew, were a large part of medical treatment.

In 1909, the station received a larger grant from Ottawa, so Dr. Watt trained his staff in the new techniques of steam sterilization. He retrofitted the shoreside fumigation building to be airtight and bought all-metal rail carts to be used for the collection of clothing bound for disinfection. He had the sewer pipes rerouted through disinfectant tanks before discharging effluent into the ocean and redesigned roof ventilators in the isolation hospitals so infectious bacteria could not escape. He also had the showers and tubs in the washhouses made more private. Dr. Watt showed a particular kindness toward Chinese immigrants who were detained at William Head, and he improved their stark quarters by replacing the hard canvas cots with steel-sprung mattresses. He improved the through-road to Victoria, and acquired a second inshore quarantine vessel, the coal-fired *Madge*. In 1910, to log the changes, he began a book of accounting records to be kept in Ottawa for the director-general of public health.

Dr. Watt grasped what the opening of the Panama Canal in 1914 would do to immigration on North America's west coast and had new nautical charts marked with the range lights and foghorn signals that were installed at the end of the peninsula. He followed the sea trials of two new, larger CPR ships, the *Empress of Russia* and the *Empress of Asia,* and understood what this whopping increase in their carrying capacity and speed would do to William Head's facilities. Dr. Watt's solution was simple. He abandoned the old daylight-only inspection rule and replaced it with a twenty-four-hour quarantine inspection policy, flooding the wharf with light from a special twenty-horsepower, shoreside generator. He had already installed a telephone line to the lighthouse at Race Rocks, which kept him abreast of the slick, new liners steaming toward William Head.[5]

Alfred Watt was at the zenith of his career, and the William Head Quarantine Station had, under his tenure, kept infectious diseases off Canada's western shores. In 1911, quarantine officials from Australia paid a special visit to learn from Dr. Watt's organizational expertise and experience. The Australians were so impressed with conditions at the station that Dr. Norris, director of quarantine for the Commonwealth of Australia, "expressed particular approval of what he saw."[6] Soon he would be asked to advise on the construction of two new inspection stations at Port Alberni and Prince Rupert.

By 1913, over 500,000 persons had been cleared through Watt's station; of those, 10,000 had been temporarily quarantined.[7] The statistics of Dr. Watt's success spoke for themselves. In 1912 alone, 161 ships arrived at the station carrying 15,762 steerage passengers, 4,637 first- and second-class cabin passengers, and 15,507 members of ships crews. In that one year, over 35,000 individuals were screened by medical officers.[8] Despite his obligations toward thousands of detainees, the wear and tear on the station's facilities, and the exhaustion of the staff, Dr. Watt was at the top of his form.

• • •

THE PRECIPICE LOOMED FOR Alfred Watt in late 1911 with the federal election and its consequent change in government. Robert Laird Borden's Conservative Party had finally ended Wilfred Laurier's fifteen-year Liberal reign. The new government did not waste any time filling Dominion appointments with loyal Conservatives. That shift in the ideology of Ottawa's power elite, and the arrival of the CPR steamship *Monteagle* two years later, pushed Dr. Alfred Tennyson Watt to the very edge of the abyss.

On March 30, 1913, the *Monteagle* arrived at William Head flying the yellow flag of quarantine and was immediately directed to the station's wharf. During the voyage, a first-class passenger named Mrs. Buchanan had caught varioloid smallpox, a less virulent but still dangerous form of the disease. Routine examinations uncovered a Chinese passenger in steerage who was also sick with the disease. Dr. Watt removed the two into separate station hospitals and detained all steerage passengers and Asiatic crew. His report was succinct: "Both passengers had come on board at Hong Kong on March 8th so that the infection presumably was from an exposure in one of the ports of Japan, possibly an ambulant case among the stevedores."[9]

Past quarantine practice had allowed those first-class passengers suspected of having had contact with the diseased to serve out their quarantine time on board ship. That enabled the privileged to avoid the less-than-luxurious conditions of shoreside detention and remain in the comfort to which they were accustomed. Dr. Watt generally opposed this policy on the grounds that healthy but suspected carriers of contagion without guards or restriction could inevitably wander freely throughout a vessel from saloon to bar, from dining room to promenade deck, picking up active infection from myriad sources. Besides, fumigating a ship with passengers underfoot was well-nigh impossible *and* dangerous.

On this particular voyage, the *Monteagle* carried 379 passengers and 261 crew, totalling 640 persons on board. Of these, 46 travelled first class, with 22 men and 24 women. There were also 290 Chinese travelling in steerage.[10] Mrs. Buchanan had mingled with many socialites, hence her movements were problematic. Dr. Watt did what was required: he emptied the ship completely and ordered the *Monteagle* cleared of all baggage and thoroughly fumigated. Two days later, with only a skeleton crew on board, the *Monteagle* cleared William Head bound for Vancouver. It arrived there on April 3, its cargo of fine silk still reeking of sulphur dioxide. Left behind were all the Chinese, most of the crew, and all those who had travelled first class. Needless to say, they were speechless at the indignity of being detained.

The *Vancouver Sun* reported that the *Monteagle* had arrived empty, but Dr. Watt's reputation had preceded the prestigious liner across the Gulf, and both he and William Head were given an especially good press. The *Sun* reported, "it is possible that the passengers will be kept at William Head until at least the end of the week . . . Dr. Watt, the quarantine officer, is said to be a good entertainer and will provide every amusement possible for the enforced white guests, who will have the run of the station golf links and other forms of outdoor amusement provided."[11] The *Daily Colonist* also reported confidently that all those on board who were detained would have an especially "pleasurable time."[12] Ironically, such good copy would later contribute to Dr. Watt's fall from grace.

• One of those left agog when the *Monteagle* departed was an especially notable member of Canadian high society. Physician and politician Dr. Judson Burpee Black had been the MP for Hants County, Nova Scotia, for twelve years, and past president of the Nova Scotia branch of the Canadian Medical Association. He was also the mayor of Windsor, Nova Scotia, for three terms and president of the Windsor Board of Trade. He and his wife were returning home from a trip around the world during which expense was of little consequence and luxury the norm. They were en route to Vancouver and thence overland to Ontario. Suddenly, among many other first-class passengers, the Blacks found themselves quarantined for fourteen days in a so-called first-class detention house at William Head with no luxuries whatsoever.

In reality, the "cabins" in the first-class quarantine house at the station were little more than barely furnished cubicles. The mandate was to prevent infectious diseases from entering a country, and their spartan fittings reflected this singular, medical objective. They were not, nor did they try to be, health spas for the rich and famous, tourist havens, or holiday resorts for travelling dilettantes. For those of the gilded age who were used to travelling first class on ships like the *Lusitania*, quarantine accommodations ashore were an insult to their person and a disgrace to their class.

Due to Dr. Watt's mass detention policy, everything at the William Head Quarantine Station was stretched beyond its limit. First-class detainees, as all others, had to undergo the dreaded disinfecting shower and daily examinations. This humiliation was further intensified when many felt ignored by Dr. Watt himself. After a week, five first-class saloon passengers, including Dr. and Mrs. Black, were distressed enough to form a protest committee. They had read the *Daily Colonist*'s sanguine promises of a "pleasurable time" at William Head and decided to go public with what was for them a more accurate view. They wrote a letter of protest to government officials in Victoria, alleging poor housing, unsatisfactory sanitation procedures, and ill treatment by its chief medical officer. They mailed a copy to Martin Burrell, the Conservative minister of agriculture in Ottawa, and sent off another to the editor of the *Daily Colonist*. Whatever the newspapers had said, they were having a most *unpleasurable* time at William Head, and the world was going to hear of it.

> The following facts regarding the disgraceful conditions of the William Head Quarantine Station will show you our lot is far from enviable. The unsuitability of the accommodation granted by the Government, its unsanitary conditions, and the tardy assistance rendered passengers and CPR officials by the Agricultural Dept., called for protests from the Monteagle passengers. An indignation meeting was therefore convened and a committee appointed to formulate

specific charges which we regrettably find necessary to bring against
Quarantine administration.[13]

• It did not take long for a determined Judson Burpee Black to file a law-
suit against Dr. Watt in the Assize Court on May 20, 1913. The man was
out for blood, claiming:

1. A quarantined passenger had escaped from the station. (He was
   recaptured.)
2. A detained passenger was allowed to meander at will outside the
   station grounds and return at his leisure.
3. A man from Victoria mixed with quarantined patients daily before
   returning home.
4. Four days before the quarantine was lifted, fourteen detainees who
   reported that their vaccination had not taken were sent to Victoria
   and allowed to travel freely.
5. Dr Watt was guilty of "unfair discrimination," in that two fer-
   vent anti-vaccinationists were allowed to travel to Victoria while
   Dr. Black and his wife were not.
6. The facilities at the station were poorly equipped and unable to
   handle such a large number of detainees.[14]

Reporters covering the story were floored; Victoria citizens were flab-
bergasted. That these charges coming from a man of such eminence as
Dr. Black were directed toward *their* Dr. Watt was unthinkable. Some of the
conditions that Judson Burpee Black had described were endemic to quarantine stations worldwide, and some were perennial concerns that the chief
medical officer had inherited from the time of his appointment. Yet, Dr. Watt
knew that some of the charges, damaging as they were, were outright lies. He
would give his honest view to the judge and use this most public occasion to
argue for improved facilities at the station, something that more recent dispatches to the new, Conservative overlords in Ottawa had failed to achieve.

On June 2, 1913, Dr. Black's condemnation of the William Head
Quarantine Station made the front page of the *Vancouver Sun,* and
Dr. Watt's leadership was front and centre:

QUARANTINE STATION COMPLAINTS CAUSE OF SERIOUS INDICTMENTS BY PASSENGERS OF MONTEAGLE.
—Facilities not in Fit State to Live In—
—Unfair Treatment on Part of Doctor is Allegation—
—Place not Sufficiently Guarded from Visitors—
—Former President of Medical Association
Will Lay Grave Charges—

My complaint is not against the station itself, though that is bad enough, and I shall take that up with Honourable Martin Burrell, Minister of Agriculture, when I reach Ottawa. My indictment is against Dr. Watt, the superintendent of the quarantine station, and I accept all responsibility for that indictment.[15]

Judson Burpee Black's vehemence toward Dr. Watt was palpable; some thought it personal.

At the hearings in Victoria, Dr. Watt defended William Head as a work in progress. Judge Moore paid a special visit to the station and verified that construction and renovation were everywhere. Station facilities had been continually updated as shown by the annual reports that Watt had submitted to Ottawa. Aroused by the unsolicited attack, Alfred Tennyson Watt initially went on the offensive.

Of the unclean bathrooms, Dr. Watt showed that at the time of the *Monteagle*'s quarantine, the bathrooms, such as they were, *were* clean: "two men had been employed all the time in cleaning the floors."[16] Of the variable water temperature, Watt showed that water for cabin and steerage detainees was abundant and heated in the same tank, and the measured temperature variant was small. He did admit, however, that Chinese detainees had used hot water to wash their dishes—something that for them was a recent luxury. Dr. Watt told the court that all station workers had been vaccinated and so were protected *and* safe. The anti-vaccinationists he had allowed into Victoria had admitted to him secretly that they *were* vaccinated two years before and therefore posed no risk. But it was true, he admitted, that one man did escape.

Dr. Watt was questioned at length regarding accommodations for detainees at William Head. His responses revealed much about the general attitude toward race and class extant in Britain and Canada at the end of the nineteenth century. The treatment of those at the William Head Quarantine Station simply revealed a wider cultural predisposition for which Dr. Watt was neither responsible nor to blame. The *Daily Times* printed the interrogation:

"How many acres of ground are there for the use of passengers?"

"Sixty acres. The seaward portion consisting of about thirty acres is for the use of the steerage people."

"What buildings are there in the steerage quarter?"

"Two, one for Chinese, and one for Japanese passengers. The Chinese building is one-storied, with three rooms, containing two large dormitories in each of which there are 96 galvanized iron beds. Meals are taken in the smaller room between the dormitories The kitchen is in the centre of the building. The greatest number [of Chinese] accommodated at any one time had been 450."

"And yet you have only accommodation for 192?"

"Most of the Chinese slept on the floor. They each have a space of two feet broad and six feet long."

"How high was the room?"

"Ten feet. The Japanese building was even smaller, being fashioned to accommodate 150 people."

"Then each man had only 120 cubic feet of air. Do you consider that sufficient?"

"It was as much as they got [in steerage] on the steamer."[17]

Accommodations for first- and second-class, largely British detainees at William Head were different. The first-class detention building in 1913 had twenty-eight seven-by-nine-foot cabins and could only accommodate fifty-four passengers. At the time of the *Monteagle*'s arrival, the first-class detention house on the station had only two drafty bathrooms, but these were being increased to eight.

At William Head, second-class passengers were housed in an old hospital building, which Watt readily admitted needed repair. The building had only twenty beds and housed those who had shared a cabin with perhaps two or three others on board. It was also used to detain members of a ship's crew. The interrogation continued:

"How many first-class passengers do the steamships usually carry?"
   "They have carried from 7 to 180 saloon passengers."
   "How many did the *Monteagle* carry?"
   "Forty-six."
   "What would you do if a ship came alongside your wharf tomorrow with 180 Saloon passengers?"
   "Some of the passengers would have to go into tents."[18]

Watt understood the inadequacy of his facilities given the burgeoning technological changes of the early twentieth century, and court records revealed he had made several appropriations to Ottawa for improved disinfecting and lavatory facilities. When asked his most serious need, Watt's reply was clear and categorical: "more accommodation!"[19]

Captain Archibald was chief of supply for Canadian Pacific Steamships, and told Judge Moore of his experiences as master of the *Empress of China* when it was detained at William Head in 1897. As required, his Chinese passengers were disembarked, but he had refused to land any first-class passengers, simply because all their bedding, crockery, utensils, *and* food came from his ship. "The great defect was that the place [William Head] was absolutely empty except for the bare boards, a few chairs and cooking stoves. Everything had to be supplied by the company."[20] In the intervening years, he believed little had changed.

Then Captain Archibald added that the "complaints of the passengers were somewhat overdrawn."[21] From his own experience, he believed "Dr. Watt and the other quarantine officials had always been most friendly and that Dr. Watt would do all that he could both for passengers and crew."[22]

Suddenly, halfway through the enquiry, Martin Burrell, federal Conservative minister of agriculture, ordered a special committee sent to William Head. Courteous and open, Dr. Watt hid nothing from their prying eyes. Much to the chagrin of Judson Burpee Black, the committee wrote, "it was indebted to Dr. A.T. Watt for the courteous manner in which he afforded opportunity to make a thorough inspection of the premises."[23]

Their report could find nothing wanting in the administration of the station, and their recommendations simply echoed Watt's desire for improved first- and second-class facilities.

James Ogden Grahame, a first-class passenger and member of the protesting committee, testified on May 30. He complained, "the bath was on the cold side and chilled us."[24] He whined that the pillowslip he had been given to hold his clothes destined for disinfection was too small, "and there was no room for my overcoat."[25] He fussed that the air in his first-class cubicle that he shared with his wife was, after thirteen days, "foul." Besides, he added, "the room was dangerous. I slipped from a stool when trying to put out the lamp . . . There was only a little 15-cent Siwash looking glass . . . and the furniture was a disgrace."[26] Grahame continued, "The authorities who built it must have known that it was not like a cabin on a ship where there are skylights."[27]

When Mr. Grahame faced enforced detention in conditions far beneath his station, he felt his place in society had been compromised and his divine right of privilege suddenly brought into question. Grahame had grown accustomed to the aristocratic excess inherent in the era of playboy-king Edward VII as manifest in the luxury liners of the *Empress* fleet, or on the *Britannic* and *Titanic*. Yet even these great liners had accommodation for steerage passengers, a feature that their counterparts in ships like the *Elizabeth and Sarah*[28] some sixty years before could only have imagined. In those days, the crossing for full-rigged ships would take one hundred days, and the vessels were little more than wholesale breeding grounds of contagion and death. Now, slick ocean steamships such as the *Lusitania* raced from Fishguard to New York in less than five days, and even the *Monteagle*, when pushed by Captain Davidson, was able to cross the Pacific in a respectable thirteen and a half days. When the *Titanic* had plummeted to the bottom of the icy Atlantic the year before, and the *Lusitania* was torpedoed a year later, Grahame's sense of invincibility and permanence had foundered. The world had changed. In 1913, James Ogden Grahame suddenly found himself shivering in a cubicle in a clapboard building with few amenities and pitiful service on the rainy edge of nowhere, and it scared him.

Not all detained first-class passengers on the *Monteagle* were as indignant or alarmed as James Ogden Grahame or Judson Burpee Black. In a letter to the minister of agriculture, passenger R.S. Kinney echoed the testimony of Captain Archibald. He revealed that the committee did not speak for him. "From a conversation I had with Dr. Black before leaving the station, I should say that the grounds of his complaint against Dr. Watt are more personal than anything else . . . Further I think that the so-called protest is more political than anything else and it has been too highly coloured."[29]

It was only when Dr. Walker and Dr. Hunter, former staff physicians at the William Head Quarantine Station, testified against Dr. Watt that the full force of this more personal agenda became known. Both Walker and Hunter felt they had been professionally slighted by Dr. Watt, and the resentment they unleashed upon their former boss had no bounds. They vilified Watt's character in open court and the bitterness of their attack caught the doctor completely off guard.

Dr. Walker was a man of facts. He had an abiding belief in the absolute supremacy of numbers and was the quintessential mad scientist. His ethical sense was simple: issues were either right or wrong, and there could be no in-between.

The pompous young physician opened his testimony with a statement completely contrary to earlier ones. From a sanitation point of view, Walker exclaimed, "The station was *absolutely bad*."[30]

Over the cynical guffaws of hardened reporters, Dr. Walker exclaimed that his opinion "was not based on existing theories but on facts that had been established experimentally."[31] Walker believed "every passenger should have an air space of 1,000 cubic feet. Taking into account the space occupied by the beds, trunks, and other articles in the 'cabins,' the air space in them thus amounted to only 102 cubic feet."[32] He went on: "Air cannot be changed more than three times in a confined space without causing a harmful draught."[33] Based upon these numbers, the "cubic contents of the cubicles were totally inadequate for the purposes for which they were intended."[34] When asked more directly if the sulphur-dioxide fumigation process or the disinfecting showers worked, not on drafts but on germs, Walker, a little taken aback, stated that these operations were "satisfactory."

Dr. Watt's solicitude would have been hard-pressed to tolerate Walker's pedantry. The amount of air space, the good doctor understood, was not the only measure of accommodation size. The harsh reality of thousands of incoming ships, many of which required quarantine, dictated more difficult decisions than the reconstruction of the universe based upon questionable numerical assumptions.

Yet, Dr. Walker claimed, too, that his superior rarely consulted him, and as assistant medical officer he felt he should have been consulted. He reiterated the tale of his discovery of two stowaways on a quarantined vessel and how he had them immediately jailed in William Head's makeshift lockup. In Walker's eyes, they had done wrong and therefore had to be punished. The fact that they were also impoverished and could not speak English did not seem to hold sway. Dr. Watt released them immediately without consultation. The William Head Quarantine Station, he knew, was not a prison but a hospital driven by the compassion inherent in a physician's Hippocratic Oath.

In Watt's eyes, Dr. Walker was a complete fool. He was also a card-carrying Conservative. He had resigned his position at William Head on December 1, 1911, a full year and a half *before* the hearings began. What had prompted the convenient resurrection of his past gripes?

Dr. Hunter replaced Dr. Walker as assistant medical officer and station bacteriologist. Ottawa's Conservative government had appointed him, and Dr. Watt had neither any say in the decision nor any power in his removal. Dr. Hunter had written to the Department of Agriculture in Ottawa and complained that his superior often dismissed him. In court, Dr. Hunter claimed he had received little training from Dr. Watt when he had first arrived, and after a month he was ignored completely. Hunter continued:

> *On Saturday afternoon, I was told that the* Monteagle *was coming in and would possibly be detained for smallpox. Early on Sunday morning I did not go on board, but waited around for something to do. The superintendent gave me no instructions. Indeed, he took no notice of me whatever. During the whole time of* Monteagle's *quarantine the only thing I was told was, "You had better look after the First-Class passengers."*[35]

As station bacteriologist, Dr. Hunter might have done a thousand tasks in preparation for an incoming vessel with smallpox on board. There was lab work to prepare and he might have begun inspections himself. It was later revealed that on May 3, a month after the landing of the *Monteagle,* another ship arrived at William Head that warranted inspection. There was a gale blowing up from Puget Sound that day, and the captain chose to stand well off the headland in Parry Bay.

The quarantine's tender, the tug *Madge,* was away at the time, and given the weather, Dr. Hunter had refused to go out to the ship in one of the station's two large man-powered lifeboats. Hunter stated, "it was scarcely that the Department of Agriculture expected its men to inspect ships in open rowboats."[36]

A delay might have been in order, but to neglect a task would have rankled Dr. Watt completely. The open rowboats were indeed large lifeboats that hung from the davits of ocean liners. They had six sets of rowlocks and were capable of carrying up to sixty people on the open sea. The lifeboats were used by workers at the quarantine station to ferry supplies over to the leper colony on Bentinck Island, across the windy mouth of Pedder Bay. Dr. Watt would have been alongside the waiting ship in a couple of pulls on the oars. More cautiously, he would have postponed the inspection until the winds settled in the evening. Dr. Hunter sat on shore and did nothing.

Then Dr. Hunter turned personal. He accused Dr. Watt of caring "more for his personal sheep-ranch than for his work in connection with issues of quarantine."[37] He alleged Watt used the station's launch to transport his prize sheep to Victoria, New Westminster, and Vancouver. But Hunter also admitted using the same launch for *his* personal jaunts to the mainland. Moreover, Dr. Watt had on one occasion lowered the payment on an invoice Dr. Hunter submitted by some sixty dollars, requesting only that he produce further receipts. Hunter never responded, but remained miffed for weeks.

It came to light that Dr. Hunter had also resigned from the William Head Station well *before* his testimony, but not before speaking with Judson Burpee Black. Dr. Black had supported Dr. Hunter in his attack against Watt, and wrote, "Dr. Watt has an assistant named Hunter, a capable young fellow, but Dr. Watt will not allow him to assist."[38] Watt responded that

Dr. Hunter's manner alternated between aggression and dismay: "He seemed to take anything I said as a direct affront. He would sulk and not speak for a long time."[39]

Hunter's mistake was his public denunciation of Dr. Frederick Montizambert, director-general of public health in Ottawa. A Liberal, Montizambert had recently visited the station and had given it a clean bill of health. Hunter stated, "They go on an inspection, they have lunch, chat, smoke, and are having a good time, and that is all."[40] Dr. Hunter's credibility diminished as the denunciation of his Liberal superiors became more hysterical. In the end, Judge Moore concurred with Dr. Watt's assessment of the station's assistant medical officer. He wrote, "Dr. Hunter adopted a hot-headed and unreasonable attitude, and seemed to have done his best to make proper co-operation between himself and his superior difficult to the point of impossibility."[41]

It was obvious. There were political forces at work to have the independent-minded Dr. Watt removed. They would succeed, but not in the way that any could have imagined.

Humiliated and fatigued, Dr. Watt considered resigning. But beyond the immediate maelstrom, he was also tortured by other demons. His eldest child, Robin, was stricken with pneumonia while away at school in Guelph, Ontario. At the time, pneumonia was often a death sentence, and Dr. Watt had spent two months away from the station in January and February 1913, agonizing over the uncertain recovery of his first son.

Then, on May 15, Watt's beloved younger brother, Hubert, died after a long struggle with cancer. Alfred was devastated. Strangely, his relationship with his brother was much like that of Lord Tennyson's relationship with his friend and mentor, Arthur Hallam.

While at Cambridge in 1827, Lord Tennyson had joined a small group of clever, young undergraduates who encouraged his poetic career. The most gifted of these was Arthur Henry Hallam, a writer with an undeniably promising future who helped Tennyson overcome his natural shyness and prodded him to publish his first volume of verse, *Poems, Chiefly Lyrical.* Tennyson idolized Hallam and introduced him to his sister Emily, to whom Hallam became engaged in 1833. When Hallam died suddenly of typhus in Vienna later that year, Lord Tennyson was completely shattered. Grief-stricken almost to the point of suicide, Tennyson recovered only after years of crafting "In Memoriam," a long, elegiac, and meditative poem evoking the death of his friend.

Dr. Alfred Tennyson Watt was shattered by the death of his dearest brother. Hubert had encouraged Alfred and offered him advice in his medical career in British Columbia. Hubert's death, coinciding with a daunting enquiry and Watt's anguish over his son, prompted Watt to write his brother a note containing two verses from "In Memoriam":

But thou and I are one in kind,
as moulded like in Nature's mint;
And hill and wood and field did print
the same sweet forms in either mind.

At one dear knee we proffer'd vows,
one lesson from one book we learn'd,
Ere childhood's flaxen ringlet turn'd
to black and brown on kindred brows.[42]

The verses distilled his feelings toward Hubert just as Tennyson's verse expressed the loss he felt over the death of Arthur Hallam.

Sadly, Alfred Tennyson Watt was unable to attend the funeral of Hubert because it was scheduled for May 20, the same day as the William Head hearings were to begin. The full force of his exhaustion overwhelmed Alfred and pulled him toward the edge. On June 21, Alfred Tennyson Watt suffered a nervous breakdown and was admitted to St. Joseph's Hospital in Victoria on the advice of his friends Dr. Robert Fraser and Dr. Hormann Robertson. They believed that only a complete rest might cure Alfred's "neurasthenia." Watt was given a room on the third floor of the hospital and assigned nurses to watch him carefully twenty-four hours a day.

It wasn't enough. In one short week, Alfred Tennyson Watt had changed from a gentleman of unfailing courtesy and kindness to a shattered shred of a man in complete collapse. Overcome by grief and guilt, he began sleepwalking. Over the course of that week, he slept, cried, and walked intermittently.

But on Saturday night, June 26, 1913, his somnambulism seemed in check after he had been given a sleeping draught. Just before 5:00 a.m. on Sunday, seeing he was in a sound slumber, the attending nurse left Watt's room for a moment for a fresh container of water. An odd noise, a slight stir of air in the hallway, caused him to pause, turn, and rush back. "The bed was empty and the curtains disarranged."[43] Alfred Tennyson Watt had simply vanished out of his third-floor window.

The *Vancouver Sun* proclaimed: "Tragic End to a Promising Career: Walks in sleep from window,"[44] while the *Victoria Daily Times* declared: "Dr. A.T. Watt Meets Death Tragically: Superintendent of Quarantine killed by fall from window of hospital. Had been suffering from Neurasthenia. Greatly worried by Death of brother, illness of son, and friction at station."[45]

Watt's broken body never lay in state. Two days later, on Tuesday, July 29, the funeral at St. Andrew's Presbyterian Church was filled to overflowing for the funeral. Hundreds more stood quietly outside. The Royal Arcanum presented a special wreath, and the church was overwhelmed with silent tributes from the Medical Association, the Seaman's Institute, the Board of Trade, cabinet ministers and staff, patients, and friends from the William Head Quarantine Hospital.

Included among the pallbearers were Alfred's old colleagues Dr. G.L. Milne and Judge Lampman. Two carriages were necessary, one for the hearse that carried the coffin, completely covered in flowers, and another for flowers alone. The slow procession of hackneys to the interment at Ross Bay Cemetery was blocks long. There, Alfred Tennyson Watt, age forty-four, was laid to rest, too late to know that Judge Moore would exonerate him completely.

Victoria knew it had lost one of its best. Most citizens understood what had caused Alfred's Watt's untimely death, and the *Victoria Daily Times* did not delay in speaking up:

DR. WATT DIED A VICTIM OF POLITICAL PERSECUTION

That the shattered condition of his nerves, which was the direct cause of his death, was due to the persecution to which he has of late been subjected, is beyond question. A valuable life has been lost to the community as a result of baseless charges, involving the integrity of one in whom a high sense of honour was combined with an unusual degree of sensitiveness . . . It is understood that since the change of administration in Ottawa [Liberal to Conservative], Dr. Watt has been somewhat hampered in the discharge of his duty by a lack of sympathetic co-operation of those employed in connection with the Quarantine Station . . . Here, we have had a case where a capable and efficient public servant, the first quarantine officer on this coast of Canada to order a steamship into quarantine, notwithstanding the protests of her commander, a man before whom, under normal conditions there would have been many years of usefulness, was driven to his death by the greed of patronage.[46]

It took a month for Dr. Watt's father to comment on the blistering editorial. Hugh Watt wrote to the editor on September 5, 1913:

The most respectful members of the Conservative Party in your city kept themselves away from the hearings, and as a matter of fact were among my son's best personal friends. I do not think that the intent of the recent commission was of a persecuting nature, but it seems to have been so manipulated to purify our Party from the baser elements that disgrace and sometimes destroy it. Those of this baser sort who were so indecently anxious to remove my son should have had greater patience, and they might have accomplished their object without having, as now, the guilt of blood upon their souls.[47]

Alfred Tennyson Watt might have fallen from grace, but class, patronage, and vengeance had fallen to a new low.

"Maud" was one of Dr. Alfred Tennyson Watt's favourite poems. It was Lord Tennyson's most cherished piece of work. A mixture of rapture and desolation, "Maud" is about a murder and the mindset of a speaker who longed for contact with what has been lost. The real truth of Dr. Alfred Tennyson Watt's life and death should be left to this excerpt from the poem:

Did he fling himself down? who knows? for a vast speculation had fail'd,
And ever he mutter'd and madden'd, and ever wann'd with despair,
And out he walk'd when the wind like a broken worldling wail'd,
And the flying gold of the ruin'd woodlands drove thro the air.

CHAPTER 8 // EAST MEETS WEST AT THE WILLIAM HEAD QUARANTINE STATION

Where are the coolies in your poem, Ned?

—Earle Birney, "Anglosaxon Street"[1]

t began innocently enough with a simple, heartfelt letter home:

My Dear Father and Mother-in-Law,

Your son-in-law left on the 5th month, 3rd day. We went aboard ship and started on our journey and travelled till the 24th. We have arrived in English Canada from where we take a train and in about 16 days we will arrive in France.

My journey has been one of peace and tranquility under the protection of the Heavenly Father and I have met with no dangers or hardships. Every day we have all we want, our eatables, clothing, and everything we want are excellent.

I hope that Mother and Father-in Law have no anxiety about me. I hope that all the members of the Church prosper and don't backslide because the Kingdom is near and we are controlled by destinies.

I thank you for taking care of my wife as she is bound to fret about my absence and furthermore present my compliments to the two families, my sisters-in-law and the eldest daughter-in-law, and I wish you a tranquil farewell.

Your Son-in-Law
Joe Hwei Chun, in reverence.[2]

Joe Hwei Chun was going to need all the faith he could muster, as he was in for the shock of his life. When he arrived at the William Head Quarantine Station on April 18, 1917, he was in transit with 2,056 of his countrymen on the *Empress of Russia,* bound for the Great War—not as a soldier exactly, but as a worker in a volunteer "clean-up" army. He had joined the Chinese Labour Corps (CLC) in Weihaiwei, China, to replace those non-combatant Allied troops in France who were being sent to the Western Front as Canadian and British casualties mounted. In total, 84,473 Chinese labourers would join the CLC and be held while in transit at the William Head Quarantine Station.[3]

They were being sent to the Ypres Salient, a curved swath of high ground from which, in 1917, the British believed they could sweep down to regain the German-occupied Belgian seaports with their deadly submarine bases in the English Channel. For the Allies, it would be a massacre with over half a million casualties in five months; villages such as Poelcappelle and Passchendaele were annihilated. It was the CLC's task to repair roads, drive supply vehicles, retrieve unexploded shells, and bury the dead. The reality meant searching for bloated and blackened corpses and rotting horse carcasses among the monstrous silhouettes and labyrinthine ruins of ancient hamlets from Lillers to Langemark.

It was a clandestine operation from the outset. From William Head, most were sent to Vancouver, transported in special trains to Halifax, and shipped to Dunkirk. The secrecy was necessary for fear that Germany might discover the enterprise, or worse, that Chinese communities across Canada would try to prevent their countrymen from continuing on. The press was allowed to report only an increase in the Chinese at William Head; they were forbidden from giving any explanation. It ended in the spring of 1920 when over forty thousand CLC volunteers were returned to China. They travelled from Halifax to William Head again in sealed trains and were processed just as quickly out of the country. Though each member of the Corps received while in France a coin-sized medal for his service to the empire, the only other official thank you was a small supper at the station for a few departing officers. Chief item on the menu was sardines on toast.[4]

In 1903, the head tax levied against Chinese immigrants had been increased from $100 to $500, but Conservative prime minister Robert Borden waived the tax for CLC members with the proviso that trains carrying them across Canada be locked and guarded. Secured railway cars each carried fifty labourers and four armed guards, while special police discreetly guarded platforms along the way.

Most were recruited from the very outer edges of China and Mongolia, and some were likely unaware of the legislated racism against Asians entering Canada. Unlike the seventeen thousand Han Chinese in the CLC, these particular "soldiers" were largely uneducated in the ways of Western culture and alien even to the rest of China. The one thing they were was huge— most were over six feet tall. Those in Joe Hwei Chun's brigade were from Shandong province in northern China; most of the others joined the CLC from Xinjiang, Gansu, and Inner Mongolia. Nellie de Bertrand Lugrin remembered seeing them at the William Head Quarantine Station, and noted, "for the most part they were an impressive-looking lot; big men, all of them, and of fine physique. Good natured too."[5]

Western missionaries and traders in the China–Mongolia hinterlands did the dirty work for the British and Chinese governments recruiting the huge numbers of men required to clear Normandy of bodies. Poverty was rife on China's northern border, so people were enticed by "a $2.50 separation allowance on leaving China and a promised one to three francs a day once they reached France."[6] The feared Chinese Provincial Police oversaw this independent fringe of Chinese/Mongolian society; their task was to muster them on China's northern frontier and transport them to the coast.

The CLC left from Weihaiwei (Port Edward), a major port city in Shandong province, which opened to the Yellow Sea. Weihaiwei was a British garrison at the time with a huge naval base and sanitarium. It had been co-opted by British colonials to counterbalance the Russian presence at nearby Lushun City (Port Arthur). In Weihaiwei, each recruit was medically examined, inoculated, given zinc-sulphate eye drops to ward off trachoma, and photographed. Their "pigtails" were removed and their heads shaved, and each had received a metal identification tag firmly fixed around their wrist. Their blue-grey uniform was a jacket containing a brigade-number and a round cap marked "CLC." Their kit was a simple bedroll, rice bowl, and tin cup. Collectively, they looked more like a penitentiary chain gang than the proud, non-combatant Allied force they were expected to become.[7]

Dr. Rundle Nelson was the chief medical officer at the William Head Quarantine Station at the time of their arrival, and it was he who had to deal with the sudden overcrowding. William Head was equipped to handle eight hundred people at best, but he knew that each chartered CPR *Empress* liner would carry far more. Increased numbers meant an increased threat of infectious disease. Dr. Nelson was on the wharf the day the *Empress of Russia* arrived at the William Head Quarantine Station and was reported to have said, "What shall we do if they have the smallpox?"[8]

One of them *did*. Nelson examined all 2,057 of them, and unceremoniously had the full complement removed from the ship and quarantined at his station for fourteen days.[9] Yet, week after week, the CPR ships *Empress of Asia, Empress of Japan,* and *Empress of Russia* disembarked thousands of new CLC recruits at the station's wharf. In July 1917, the Chinese Labour Corps had already swelled to over thirty thousand men. The Canadian Militia took official charge of the corps as they landed and created a fenced-off "coolie camp." The CLC were accommodated in army bell tents right on the doorstep of William Head, and the 5th British Columbia Company of the Royal Canadian Garrison Artillery immediately took over military discipline.

The artillery made one in every twenty members of the corps wear an armband designating a corporal's rank, and it was through these intermediaries that information regarding camp rules and routines was supposed to be disseminated. But this top-down, authoritarian model was alien to the self-reliant nomads of the Mongolian borderlands, and as conditions deteriorated at the quarantine station with the spring rains, discipline among the rank-and-file plummeted. Even with increasing punishment, their survival instinct readily eclipsed the corps' requirement for order. Most were used to the autonomy and freedom of the China/Mongolia plateau, where they would not kowtow to the southern Chinese overlords.

By October 1917, the rains began in earnest. With thousands of men arriving and departing at all hours, the grounds of the William Head

Quarantine Station soon became a quagmire. To remain dry in their tents, members of the corps "helped themselves to anything which would keep them off the wet ground, including doors of buildings, and entire walls and roof of the blacksmith's shop."[10] John Weir, a pioneer in Metchosin, complained bitterly from his nearby farm about the "Chinese soldiers." Often, he saw groups of them tramping through his property, removing fence rails for firewood and stealing vegetables for food.[11]

The William Head Peninsula is defined on its south side by Pedder Bay where, for generations, indigenous peoples fished and made a life. Here, too, a small settlement of Chinese workers had taken root, many of whom had helped construct the Canadian Pacific Railway. They had discovered, too late, that the CPR would renege on its promise to repatriate its Chinese workers, and being unable to afford to return home with what they had saved from their meagre wages, many migrated to the coast. Seeking respite from the overt racism in Victoria, some moved to the Aboriginal settlement at Pedder Bay where they interacted amicably with the Natives and pulled a good living from the sea. Several CLC members escaped the station and joined the small settlement on the bay. It was said they could earn far more fishing than they could in the killing fields of northwest Europe.

Real escapes were few, but there was one that turned out to be as humorous as it was inept. One particular gentle giant who was less interested in fishing than in the lights, music, and opium alleys of Victoria's Chinatown made a dash for it. However, like so many of his comrades, he was over six feet tall. Victoria constables readily found him towering above the others in Fan Tan Alley and promptly escorted him back to the quarantine station, where he rejoined his battalion and was sent off to Panama, bound for Britain, on the next ship.

To curtail the growing unrest, the artillery created Chinese work gangs who did laundry, cut firewood for the station, tended its vegetable and flower gardens, and made repairs to station facilities. Even in the evenings they dug trenches, dugouts, and emergency gun pits, which made some suspect that the promise of a non-combative role in France may not have been the whole truth.

The more stoic were encouraged by station officials to engage in their traditional arts and crafts. Nellie de Bertrand Lugrin reported after seeing them during a visit:

They spent hours making what they termed "pictures." They would
build a platform of rock and earth about eight by ten feet, level the
top and construct the picture. It was meant to represent a [Chinese]
story or a play, and they made it by using pebbles, bits of coloured glass,
flower blossoms and tiny shrubs. The children [of the station's staff]
were delighted with their handiwork.[12]

These life-size dioramas were strategically placed throughout the grounds of the quarantine station.

The CLC members also seemed to adore the children of station employees, and made them and their families small woven baskets and other gifts. Homesick, they watched the children play, and when they could, taught them the rudiments of their language. Wary but indulgent, Garrison Artillery continued with its compulsory afternoon military drill. As the many brigades reluctantly paraded around the grounds, they were often followed by playful, dancing children, chanting in Hamelin fashion, "one-two, one-two" in a Cantonese/Mongolian mix.

On one occasion, a five-year-old daughter of a station family went missing. Lungrin remembered, "She was a beautiful little child, with golden, curly hair, blue eyes and beloved by everyone."[13] Some suspected certain corps members. Yet, ocean currents swept around the headland and cougars lurked in the woods. Frantic, the station staff searched the grounds for the missing girl to no avail. In desperation, over two thousand CLC members were called in to help. For over two hours there was nothing, then shortly after noon, the little girl walked out of one of the buildings, "hair rumpled, and rubbing her eyes. She had crawled into a clothes chute and taken a long, long nap."[14] She was greeted with as much laughter and tears by the Mongolians, who spotted her first, as by her overjoyed parents.

That assistance cemented the bond between CLC soldiers and officials at the station, and it soon spread beyond its gates. The families of Victoria's elite were invited to William Head, and they, too, were thrilled by the friendly Mongolians. Mrs. Frederica Rockhill, daughter of Dr. Nelson, recalled, "Frequently the [quarantine] officers would invite prominent ladies from Victoria to come and see some of the crafts the coolies made, and quite a number would supply silks and embroidery threads and put in orders for cushion covers or etched brass shells."[15] Mrs. Rockhill bought an etched brass shell-casing from CLC member No.132.

• • •

THE VAST MAJORITY OF the corps were cleared with dispatch at William Head and transported to Vancouver, where they faced an eight-day train journey across the country to Halifax followed by an equally long ocean passage to Southampton. Others left the station for Britain by ship, including the *Empress of Asia,* which sailed regularly for Liverpool through the Panama Canal. The corps were ferried across the English Channel to France, where they disembarked on the beaches at Dunkirk.

It did not take long for German intelligence to find out about the scheme, and the Dunkirk unloading came under attack in September 1917. Twenty-seven members of the CLC were cut down on the French beach where they had just landed.

Once in France, the CLC fell under the stern hand of British military discipline. They were formed into companies of 500 men—476 Chinese, plus 24 British officers and Chinese NCOs. As at William Head, the men were not assigned any real military rank but designated as "class one gangers, class two gangers, and class three gangers."[16] The hardships they endured at William Head over the lack of food had taught them that military discipline could be challenged. Some Chinese soldiers went on strike in Normandy over a cut in their supply of rice, and it soon spread to mass demonstrations and violence.

In late fall of 1917, British Military Police broke up several brawls between factions within the CLC. In October, police wounded five Chinese labourers over a "disciplinary matter," and on Christmas Day of 1917, the Royal Welsh Fusiliers were ordered to break up a mutiny of a company who simply refused to work in the dangerous war zones. Nine Chinese workers were shot dead and many more were imprisoned or court-martialled. According to the Commonwealth War Graves Commission records, "between 1918 and 1920, ten Chinese Labour Corps volunteers were shot by military firing squads."[17]

Most peace-loving Chinese volunteers shrank in horror from the violence of the First World War. They were promised non-combatant duties, but that covenant was as hollow as the promise of sufficient food at William Head. The British Army could not be blamed entirely for this, as all of northern France and parts of Belgium came under fire from German heavy artillery or aircraft. From Passchendaele to Le Hamel, serial bombing by the new German Air Force massacred thousands of citizens, soldiers, and Chinese volunteers alike.

Sergeant Archie Wills from Victoria had joined up as soon as the call came in 1914. Before he was sent to the Western Front, he had heard of the Chinese Labour Corps being mobilized at the William Head Quarantine Station. By 1918, he was an artillery platoon commander, and was directed to dig gun pits near Arras in preparation for a German offensive. He made a gun pit from an abandoned garbage dump, and dug in for the duration of his assignment. In his diary, he wrote:

> Just as we were spreading our blankets one night, in through our only entrance barged half a dozen Chinese, some of whom had been at the William Head Quarantine Station . . . It was quite evident that they had the "wind up," and were astonished at the violence of the exploding shells above them.[18]

The CLC company had been "ordered close to the Front to aid in new construction work."[19] Sergeant Wills gave them temporary shelter, but during a lull in the conflagration, they made a dash to a nearby larger crater. Days later, members of the same corps were forced to clear the bodies of those under Wills's command. Somehow, Sergeant Wills survived and after the war returned to William Head to look for any of the Chinese labourers he had befriended that awful night. He found none.

The Commonwealth War Graves Commission recorded some two thousand deaths among the CLC during the Great War. Most of the dead were buried in unmarked graves in cemeteries in northern France and Belgium. Anonymous white military headstones offered little solace to a saddened wanderer, their brief inscriptions reading only, "A noble duty bravely done."[20] Without some sort of religious faith, Joe Hwei Chun, if he wasn't killed outright somewhere east of Noyelles-sur-Mer, would surely have been driven completely out of his mind.

•••

WITH THE CESSATION OF hostilities in 1918, the Allies wasted no time in shipping the CLC force back to the Coolie Repatriation Camp at William Head. The CLC arrived to find beefed-up security. Barbed wire and heavily armed guards "prevented them from being overcome with the attractions of Canada."[21] Demonstrators were jailed while British biplanes circled above their heads and took photographs. In January 1919, with eight thousand returned to William Head, there was a full-scale riot over the appalling conditions, but it came to nothing. The inmates "were rounded up and herded back at bayonet point."[22] Percy Gray, chief steward at the William Head Quarantine Station, called in the navy. A destroyer escort was sent up from Esquimalt, and stood by in Pedder Bay. It was said that troops fired a couple of shells over the station to deter further violence.[23]

Some Canadian militiamen at William Head showed more compassion. Sergeant John W. Thompson was asked by his commanding officer on one occasion to report on a "coolie" who had been seen out of bounds. Thompson investigated. Near the wharf he found a "large number gesticulating frantically and ejaculating vociferously, a circumstance which interested me to such an extent that I, too, joined the procession to ascertain the meaning of their perturbation.[24] There, he saw the group pulling a huge North Pacific octopus from the water. Thompson estimated it weighed more than 150 pounds. "It had wrapped its tentacles around the leg of the suspected Chinaman, and was attempting to pull him into the sea. Were it not for the unflinching effort of the poor soul's countrymen, he would have undoubtedly been dragged down into the deep."[25] Thompson helped them carry the grasping cephalopod to the wharf and in short order, it was dispatched into a large metal pot to become a fabulous feast of dim sum of steamed octopus, garlic, and taro root. Was Sergeant Thompson offered a sampling of the banquet? He made no reference to it in his report.

For all the horror they experienced abroad, a few CLC soldiers were determined to remain in Canada, and one escaped from William Head in 1919, attracting a great deal of public attention.

Fred Baker, a local Victoria baker, had been arrested and charged with "aiding and abetting a Chinaman to enter Canada in defiance of the Chinese

Immigration Act."[26] One day, while delivering goods to the William Head Quarantine Station, Fred met Chang Pai Ho in the camp canteen. The man was educated and spoke French, as did Fred, and they struck up a conversation. Chang Pai told Fred that he did not wish to return to China.

Fred Baker left and returned later in his own automobile. Chang Pai Ho made it to his car and was told "to lay flat on the floor of the car in order to escape detection in passing the sentry."[27] In Victoria, Baker provided Chang Pai Ho with a hotel room, money, and a job. In due course, both men were arrested, but the judge, much to the consternation of many Victoria citizens, threw the whole case out of court. "Chinese coolies who pass through Canada en route from France to their native land cannot be considered immigrants," he ruled. "As such they did not come from within the classes of prohibited persons."[28] He also stated that during the war, many "illegal" acts were done, and this case was one such example. Fred Baker was free to go. Chang Pai Ho, unfortunately, did not get a second chance. He was returned to China on the next ship.

• • •

CANADA SIMPLY WANTED THE whole episode of the Chinese Labour Corps to be over as quickly as possible. In March 1920, the last Mongolian was sent home. His repatriation was noted in the *Daily Province:*

BIGGEST CHINK ON MS *DOLLAR*
—Coolie Giant Returning to Tsingtau—

The Canadian Robert Dollar Company's largest steamship, the M.S. *Dollar* sailed from William Head on Saturday afternoon with the largest load of coolies and the largest coolie that ever left the coast. When the big vessel put to sea, Captain Abernethy had 4306 coolies on board including one placid Oriental who stood seven feet six inches in his socks, and weighed over 300 pounds. Very rapid work was done in loading the *Tsingtau Contingent*. The first man went up the gangway at 9:00 am, and the last passed over the rail three hours and ten minutes later. The last load of coolies will be taken on the *Bessie Dollar* on Saturday. There are 1400 of them, and they include the last contingent from overseas that was held here some days because it was feared they might create trouble at the William Head barracks.[29]

By April 1920, the Coolie Repatriation Camp at William Head was closed, and its commandant, Lieutenant-Colonel Milne, demobilized the regiment. The CPR steamships the *Empress of India, Empress of Japan, Empress of Asia* and *Monteagle* transported over forty thousand Chinese back to their Asian homeland. Others had been sent home directly from France. Dismissed and forgotten by most, the William Head Quarantine Station did provide their "officers," with a farewell supper.[30]

• • •

SOME SIXTY YEARS BEFORE the CLC arrived at William Head, the Chinese in Canada had already become the victims of institutional racism. In 1858, four thousand Chinese rushed to the sandbars of the Fraser River with other gold seekers from California. Mining companies only allowed them to work the bars vacated by white employees and most prospectors forcibly tried to keep them below Yale. At Bancroft it was reported that the Chinese were in league with Natives and had sold them ammunition. Poll-tax legislation, launched against them in 1860, set the tone for more dire things to come.

Considered useful to the development of western Canada, but undesirable as citizens, they were "shanghaied" in the thousands to construct the western portion of the Canadian Pacific Railway. In 1885, the poll tax was $50; by 1903, it was $500. Since 1875, British Columbia had been quietly passing increasingly restrictive legislation. "Oriental" immigrants were forbidden to work in underground mines, prohibited from holding public works jobs, excluded from homes for the aged, banned from using Crown lands, and, of course, not allowed to vote. Three years after the CLC was sent home, the Chinese Immigration Act of 1923 barred Chinese people from entering Canada entirely.

The ramifications of these policies against Chinese communities in British Columbia were enormous. Effectively shut out of higher-paying jobs the Chinese were reduced to being second-class citizens. They took refuge as cooks, waiters, and laundry workers. Their communities were predominantly male, with a ratio of 2,800 men to 100 women until well after the Second World War.[31] Concubines were not uncommon; mixed marriages were virtually non-existent. Single men and lonely married men gravitated to opium, squalor, and disease. It is not surprising that policies of public health in British Columbia in the late nineteenth century reflected this legislated racism by linking leprosy to the Chinese, perpetuating the anti-Asian feeling.

Nowhere was this racialized disease policy more manifest than in the treatment of the Chinese lepers on D'Arcy Island. Leprosy was never epidemic in British Columbia; more Chinese died of smallpox and tuberculosis than of leprosy in BC. Yet the aphorism that the Chinese were a "leprous race" became ingrained at all levels of the provincial psyche. Rumours of leprosy in Chinese communities abounded in British Columbia during the last years of the nineteenth century. On April 5, 1882, the body of a Chinese labourer was found in a rooming house in New Westminster. It had been burned to hide evidence of leprosy. In 1890, another Chinese leper was first placed in one of Victoria's three quarantine houses, then moved to D'Arcy Island where he was abandoned. In 1891, when Victoria medical officers detected several cases of leprosy among the city's Chinese inhabitants, E.W. Foster, a Victoria justice of the peace, wrote, "Chinese lepers were allowed to go about the city and in consequence the public health was endangered."[32]

Foster's outrage soon reached other parts of Canada, as seen in a report from the *Toronto Mail* on February 6, 1891, which wrote: "Word comes from British Columbia that cases of leprosy are being discovered among the Chinese there, and that the loathsome disease is being communicated to the Indians."[33]

In May 1891, Victoria Council constructed an isolated leper lazaretto on D'Arcy Island. Five lepers were sent there under the auspices of the Victoria Board of Health. Located on the eastern edge of Haro Strait and separated from Vancouver Island by the four kilometres of Cordova Channel, D'Arcy

Island lay some forty kilometres from Victoria. The D'Arcy Island lazaretto "concretized pervasive ideas of the Chinese as a leprous race and more importantly, reinforced public and governmental opinion that Chinese immigration needed to be curtailed."[34] In 1899, the *Daily Colonist* reported, "These lepers are all Chinamen. If the people of British Columbia had their own way, Chinamen would be excluded from the provinces."[35] It took only eight years for a policy of exclusion to become a policy of deportation. The humane caring for the sick had been compromised; public health and ideas about race had become one.

Though the Victoria Council described conditions on D'Arcy Island as "comfortable," the reality was entirely different. The first lepers exiled there lived in a line of huts constructed under one roof. Each hut had only a bed, a stove, and a chair. When able, patients were expected to cook for themselves. Supplies arrived four times a year and included food, clothing, Chinese whiskey, opium, and, on occasion, coffins. Victoria medical officers visited irregularly, and when they did, only a few mentioned the appalling conditions. Dr. Duncan, chief medical officer at William Head, visited D'Arcy Island in 1897 and reported only the barest of facts: "1897. Visited D'Arcy four times in the year. Eight lepers. All Chinese. One death."[36]

Less than a year later, Dr. Duncan was urging that all Chinese immigrants entering British Columbia, regardless of health, should undergo personal disinfection at the William Head station, something not required of any other immigrant group. For fourteen years, 1891 to 1905, even the simplest medical treatment of chaulmoogra oil was not provided for the island leper colony. Not surprisingly, by 1895 the mortality rate on the D'Arcy Island was 60 percent.[37]

The compulsory isolation and abandonment of the Chinese lepers on D'Arcy Island was a response to British Columbia's view of itself as a white, Anglo-Saxon, Protestant society. The Chinese language, culture, and cosmology did not fit within the colonial vision of the respectable white settler, and this construct was further enhanced by the hideousness of leprosy itself. The racial prejudice readily translated into inadequate financial support, and the resentment the Chinese lepers had for those who had abandoned them was palpable. When a white man was isolated on the island with them and died shortly thereafter, it was reported that "the Chinese shunned him so completely that they would not even bury his body."[38]

During the thirty-one-year period that D'Arcy Island operated, forty-three of the forty-nine men banished to the island were Chinese.[39] The others were German, Russian, Japanese, Chilean, Doukhobor, and Jewish. They, too, were racialized on the basis of not being WASPs, and were believed to have caught "Chinese leprosy" from living like or among the Chinese. Fear and resentment led to the view of "Chinese leprosy" as a highly communicable disease, thus legitimizing a public health policy of isolation and abandonment.

The truth is that the disease is not very contagious at all, but epidemiologists were unclear about its spread and mode of transmission.[40] Many believed the disease was transmitted by sexual contact. Dr. John Helmcken was among the first physicians in Victoria who questioned its progression. Speaking before the Royal Commission on Chinese Immigration, he said, "Leprosy is not considered a contagious disease . . . it is more or less hereditary . . . people residing and cohabiting with them [lepers] do not take the disease."[41] Helmcken was half-right in his views of its contagion, but wrong in the details of its transmission.

It is now believed leprosy is spread by prolonged close contact with another infected person. The long incubation period varies from two to ten years, and this makes the disease difficult to track. The rod-shaped bacterium *Mycobacterium leprae* had only just been isolated by Gerhard Armauer Hansen in Norway in 1873, and its symptoms and invidious progress still challenged science. The bacterium was so much like other bacilli that microscopic identification alone was insufficient in determining its presence. According to Dr. Nelson, chief medical officer at William Head during the 1920s, "The only positive way of identification [of the disease] was to inject a rabbit. If you got no results, you could be pretty sure that it was leprosy. But if it was tuberculosis, it would show up in the animal."[42] Nelson believed that leprosy was not a zoonotic disease and hence unable to cross the animal–human barrier. However, more recent studies have shown that the armadillo *is* susceptible to it.

Leprosy is chronic and produces postulating boils, and if left untreated, it results in permanent damage to the skin, eyes, and limbs. *Mycobacterium leprae* thrives in the cooler areas of the body, so the nose, eyes, ears, hands, feet, and testicles often become infected first. Damage to the nervous system ensues; the subsequent insensitivity to pain in various parts of the body results in collateral injury as the victim has no means of monitoring sensation. Hard, painless lumps often appear on the backs of hands or on the soles of feet. As the disease progresses, the fingers and toes curl inward, grasping becomes difficult, and walking becomes impossible. Other disfigurations include skin lesions and open sores that do not heal. Labelled "unclean" in many parts of the world, lepers "were forced to live in seclusion until they died."[43] In India today, there are more than 1,000 leper colonies, and in 2011, the World Health Organization (WHO) reported 219,000 new cases worldwide.

Public fear of and private disgust at the lepers on D'Arcy Island remained even as increasing head taxes reduced the numbers of Asian immigrants who entered the country. In 1899, Victoria medical officer Dr. Fraser urged the Canadian government to take over the expense of the colony "in the misbegotten hope that the handful of BC lepers would then be transported to the federal leprosarium at Tracadie, New Brunswick."[44] Dr. Fisher, head of the quarantine service in Ottawa, firmly rejected British Columbia's repeated pleas for aid. He claimed that although the island facility was dismal and the lepers unfortunate, "they were still better off than the lepers in China."[45]

In 1905, the province of British Columbia assumed the management of D'Arcy Island, and with head-tax monies it received, it reimbursed the City of Victoria for its previous costs. Improvements to the accommodations were made, and fresh vegetables were delivered monthly. Yet, during the short, eighteen-month period of provincial responsibility, the lepers on D'Arcy Island still did not receive any meaningful medical treatment.

When the federal government passed the Leprosy Act in 1906, Ottawa was already receiving a head tax from each new Chinese immigrant that was ten times higher than it was in 1885. With this revenue, Ottawa could assume responsibility for the lazaretto on D'Arcy Island. Under federal control, and with Chinese money in hand, medical treatment for the eight marooned lepers began in 1907.[46] But Ottawa's agenda for the lepers was non-existent.

As early as February 1893, Dr. MacNaughton-Jones had proposed to the federal minister of agriculture that "they could probably get rid of the Chinese lepers if a ship could be found that would take them back to Hong Kong."[47] A decade later, a more enlightened director-general of public health, Dr. Montizambert, suggested that the leper colony ought to become part of the William Head Quarantine Station and be housed in the abandoned Albert Head facility. There, the lepers would receive proper medical attention and more humane treatment. Legislators balked at Montizambert's plan. For the moment, deportation was cheaper.

Changes in immigration legislation by 1907 allowed for the deportation of foreigners deemed "unfit." Such legislation still exists and is used to rid Canada of illegal immigrants and criminals. To deport those who had simply become sick was, even in 1907, quite a stretch, yet, in March of that year, eight afflicted Chinese left Canada for a Presbyterian mission and leper hospital in Canton. Canada had promised each of them $300 in gold upon their departure. In all, twenty-one men on the island were legally deported between 1907 and 1917.[48] After 1917, immigration law changed such that it was no longer possible to summarily deport those who had lived in Canada for at least five years.

Dr. Montizambert's view eventually prevailed, and plans were undertaken in 1906 to transport the lepers from D'Arcy Island to the unused facility at Albert Head. When news of this plan became public, Victoria citizens were beside themselves. On July 21, 1906, one angry resident wrote:

> To the Editor.—Sir, the citizens cannot too soon bestir themselves in the matter of the proposal to transfer the leper station from D'Arcy Island to Albert Head. There can be no doubt that the carrying out of such a project, no matter how slight might be the risk of contagion, would seriously cripple the expansion of Victoria . . . The country is surely large enough to afford the Minister of Agriculture

a wide choice of other sites without thrusting upon the Capital such an adjunct as this.

—S.G. Fetherston.[49]

Fetherston's letter fostered a petition of some two hundred signatures from the residents of nearby Esquimalt and Metchosin. It was presented to Premier McBride in late July 1906, and the proposal was stopped dead in its tracks.

On April 1, 1917, D'Arcy Island's caretaker died and was not replaced. In 1924, the federal government closed the lazaretto for good. Interestingly, the closing occurred just one year after the Chinese Exclusion Act became law.[50]

In 1924, the Department of Health moved the six remaining Chinese lepers to a new lazaretto on Bentinck Island. Its location off Rocky Point was just over a kilometre from the William Head Quarantine Station, and the new colony soon gained the complete support of more enlightened medical officials.

Bentinck Island lies so close to the tip of Rocky Point, the southernmost point of Vancouver Island, that it is said that the deer are able to make their way to it across a narrow channel to it at low tide. Shaped something like a cloverleaf, Bentinck Island has three bays and several protected little coves. On its northwest side facing Eemdyk Passage, there is a private sandy beach, and at high tide the sea flows swiftly through the channel, its kelp beds hiding many submerged rocks. Near the beach is the jetty to which a launch could be secured after motoring over from the William Head Quarantine Station. A flat, slightly open shelf of land slightly beyond the jetty provided just enough room for the residences of the caretaker, the nurse, and the patients themselves.

• • •

BORN IN ODESSA, UKRAINE, in 1876, Abraham Bercovich was the son of a Jewish peasant. At eighteen, with limited prospects, Abraham joined the imperial Russian army. For the next ten years he lived the unhealthy life of a soldier, was involved in a costly war against Japan, and felt the rumblings of revolution. When he heard of mass protests against

Czar Nicholas II evolving into full-blown labour strikes and a new ideology strengthening the workers' resolve for change, he knew that he may someday be on the losing side of a violent revolution. Although the czar would cling to power for another twelve years, Abraham Bercovich could see that the days of Russian imperial rule were numbered, and in late 1905, he fled to Canada with his young bride. He found work in one of Winnipeg's many dairies, built a home, and raised a family in this ethnically diverse, Jewish-friendly prairie city.

Bercovich first noticed scars on his feet in 1913. By 1921, the scars had failed to heal and had turned into hard nodes. Telltale lumps appeared on his hands, and lesions covered his face and left eyebrow. Dr. Gordon Bell diagnosed him with leprosy in 1925 and suggested he be sent to William Head.[51]

Just getting there was a chore, as the Canadian National Railway (CNR) "demanded that he must pay $1,343.75 for 25 first-class tickets, the cost of one entire colonist railway car, and a $15 follow-up fumigation fee after the transcontinental train reached Vancouver."[52] When he finally arrived with his wife, the couple initially moved into the quarantine station together. But as the disease progressed, he was moved to the leper colony on nearby Bentinck Island. In 1926, Abraham Bercovich was the ninth leper in the colony. Seven of the others were from China and one was from Russia.

For four years, Abraham was treated orally with chaulmoogra oil, but the vile black drops caused indigestion, vomiting, and gastric ulcers. Then he was given sodium cyanoacetate, or isoniazid, which Dr. Brown believed to be less poisonous. It did no good. Abraham Bercovich died of complications from advanced leprosy on February 15, 1928, and "his body was returned to Winnipeg in a metal-lined, sealed coffin."[53]

When Dr. Jenkins took over from Dr. Brown as chief medical officer at William Head in 1939, he inherited Brown's frustration over the limited benefit of chaulmoogra oil. He wrote, "it was absolutely no good at all and so it was a hopeless type of feeling that accompanied the leper who went into Bentinck."[54] He empathized with the cloistered, wasted lives of the lepers. "Man's inhumanity to man in the treatment of leprosy since pre-biblical times has been a cruel thing and there was a time when lepers were burned to death. I am not sure that our total policy of isolation was much better."[55]

Dr. Jenkins initiated regular twice-weekly visits to Bentinck Island and became fully involved in the care and treatment of the lepers. "I'd go on a Monday and my assistant would go on a Friday or Saturday to see they were well cared for and well housed."[56] He upgraded living conditions, with each patient receiving a small, detached, clapboard cottage—some even boasted a tiny porch. Heated by a wood stove in the fall and winter, each house had a bedroom, a kitchen/living area, and plentiful water. The lepers were encouraged to remain positive by tending their own vegetable garden, doing their own cooking, and, on occasion, hosting dinner parties for other inmates. Some even raised chickens. They painted the trim on their neat little homes and took pride in tending the flowerbeds that bordered the pathways between the cottages and the jetty.

As blindness and other chronic infirmities made these tasks impossible as the disease progressed, Dr. Jenkins hired a full-time caregiver. A leper in remission, the caregiver cooked and cleaned for those disabled on Bentinck from 1939 until the colony closed in 1957.

Nurse Dorothy Fairweather also worked and lived among the lepers on Bentinck Island for fifteen years, from 1934 to 1949. Her husband, Captain Neville Fairweather, lived at the nearby quarantine station with the couple's two children and ran one of the station's workboats. Encouraged by Dr. Jenkins's more open visitation policy, Neville visited his wife regularly. Though it was against the rules, their children visited on weekends. Captain Fairweather was also a botanist, and classified all the wildflowers on Bentinck, discovering over one hundred species.

Dorothy Fairweather turned her respectable one-and-a-half-storey home on Bentinck into a centre that welcomed the lepers, and she modified a room in the caretaker's house into the island's medical station. In 1931, there were nine patients housed comfortably in the Bentinck Island lazaretto. Ten years later, Dr. Jenkins had electrical power connected to each cabin and installed a telephone in the nurse's cottage.

When Dorothy Fairweather retired, she was replaced by nurse Evelyn Worsley. She lived on Bentinck for eight years, until the colony closed.

Evelyn admitted to taking the job when others were afraid to apply, and she, too, came to understand the need to expunge the lepers' isolation that came with a life of exile. She brightened each cottage with colourful curtains and cushions, and had the caretaker paint water barrels and benches a cheerful red. She encouraged the lepers to play the hand-cranked Edison gramophone in the medical station and experiment with the new-fangled radio. She taught them English, board games, and cards, and encouraged hobbies such as painting, carving, and whittling. She also insisted that the lepers regularly mail parcels home and saw to it that all outgoing gifts, such as knitted items and model boats, were properly fumigated at the quarantine station before being sent on.

Dr. Jenkins also visited other, more progressive leper facilities in North America for updates in leprosy treatment. He went to the leprosarium in Tracadie-Sheila, New Brunswick, which housed over 330 lepers by 1920. He observed the research being conducted at the National Leprosarium in Carville, Louisiana, and adopted some of the treatments at the leper colony on Bentinck Island. He was one of the first physicians in Canada to try Diasone (diamino-diphenyl-sulfone, or DDS), a new sulfa drug developed in Britain and clinically tested on lepers in America.

• During the mid-1940s, the Diasone treatment on Bentinck Island was so successful that Dr. Jenkins released four lepers. He wrote, "Just three months after the first sulfa pills were administered, we witnessed dramatic results. One elderly patient, unable to walk when he was first admitted, recovered the use of his legs after sulfa treatment."[57] Dr. Jenkins organized individual monthly packets of sulfa medication and sent them to the medical authority in those communities where his patients moved. Through Dr. Jenkins's work, the Bentinck Island leper facility became well known, and by the mid-1940s the lazaretto had grown to house 22 patients.

Dr. Jenkins encouraged visitors to Bentinck Island, though touching was to be kept to a minimum and children were not allowed. One of the first visitors was Evelyn Jenkins, the doctor's wife. Initially, she was afraid to put her hand on the gangway railings that lead from the jetty to the shore, but as time passed and she remained healthy, Mrs. Jenkins became as much a fixture on the island as her husband.

The Reverend Harold Michael Bolton of St. Mary the Virgin Anglican Church in Metchosin made weekly trips to Bentinck Island for some thirty years. By 1940, Lim Yuen of the Chinese Mission in Victoria was making regular visits. In May 1948, a journalist from *Maclean's* magazine, visited the colony. His article generated considerable international interest, and several readers from as far away as Los Angeles sent the lepers gifts. In January 1952, a fourteen-year-old Chinese leper responded so well to treatment that he received $100 from the petty officers' mess at HMCS Naden for his future education. The *Daily Colonist* reported, "Jackie received his navy visitors like old friends. He told them how he planted potatoes a day or so ago in his small garden, and how his nine chickens were not laying because of the cold weather," all in perfect English.[58]

Two years later, in January 1954, in response to a request by nurse Worsley, soldiers from the 119th Ack-Ack Battery of the Royal Canadian Corps of Signals donated a new, twenty-one-inch television set and exterior aerial to the lepers on Bentinck. "We all agreed that it was a splendid idea, all the officers, warrant officers, NCOs and men of the battery have volunteered to contribute."[59] The examination room in the caretaker's cottage soon became the island's new "theatre."

There was only one dark note, and that occurred on Bentinck Island in 1926. One of the lepers who had previously lived on D'Arcy Island killed another Chinese patient in a violent outburst. One of the cabins was turned into a makeshift jail to hold the distraught perpetrator until police arrived. In the next thirty years, the "jail" on Bentinck Island was never used again.

By 1947, there were only three lepers left on Bentinck Island. One was a middle-aged woman who had been a missionary in Africa. Another was a middle-aged, one-eyed Chinese male who knew little English. The third was "Mike," a twenty-nine-year-old Japanese Canadian who studied carpentry by mail.[60] In 1952, the missionary was released. She wrote of her time on Bentinck, "My friends have stood by me. They think more of me now than they ever did. But some acquaintances will not visit my family any longer because I am here. The disease itself is not so bad, nor is the isolation on beautiful Bentinck Island. It is being cast out that hurts. If people took a different, more sensible attitude to our disease, there is no reason why we should not live in an institution like a tuberculosis sanitarium."[61]

• With changes in medication following the use of sulfa drugs and antibiotics in the late 1940s, deaths from leprosy were all but eliminated. One eighty-three-year-old patient who had been transferred to Bentinck Island from D'Arcy Island died in 1946 of old age. Another died in 1956 at the age of seventy-six. Although his disease had been arrested, he chose to remain on Bentinck because he had no other suitable place to go. He was buried along with twelve others in the small graveyard located in a meadow near the centre of the small island. The Bentinck Island lazaretto had become his home.

At the end of 1956, those few lepers still requiring treatment were transferred to the Hôtel-Dieu de Saint-Joseph de Tracadie in New Brunswick. The official closing of the leper colony on Bentinck Island occurred on October 1, 1957. After its closure, the island was offered as a rental property "for the ridiculous sum of $40 per month."[62] There were no takers. Two years later, the federal government signed the island over to the Department of National Defence, which used the land for training purposes. It remains under their jurisdiction.

In the 1980s, a team from the Department of National Defence (DND) did an inventory of the existing buildings on Bentinck Island, which they felt deserved documenting for historical purposes. Many of the structures of the colony had been demolished, and what was left was overgrown. Two buildings, the nurses' house and one leper cabin, remained intact. The nurses' house was maintained for a time in its original shape, but the leper cabin was vandalized and eventually torn down. The graveyard, the final resting place of some of the colony's inhabitants, was enclosed by a fence by the DND in 1983. Above the graves, anonymous crosses were installed. Bentinck Island remains closed to the public today.

In October 2000, Victoria mayor Alan Lowe and author C.J. Yorath unveiled a small plaque in remembrance of the Chinese lepers who were abandoned on D'Arcy Island. Although the leper colony on Bentinck Island was a far more humane and successful treatment centre, it has not been memorialized.

Chinese steerage passengers detained at William Head Station in 1917.

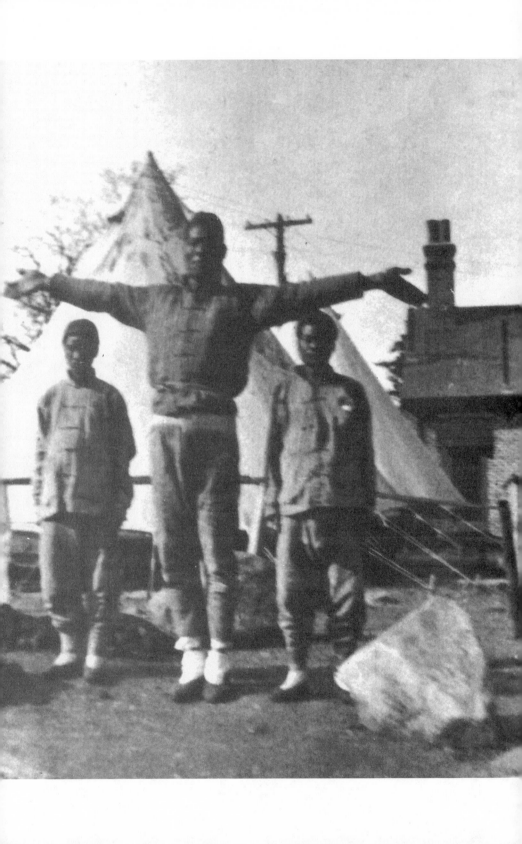

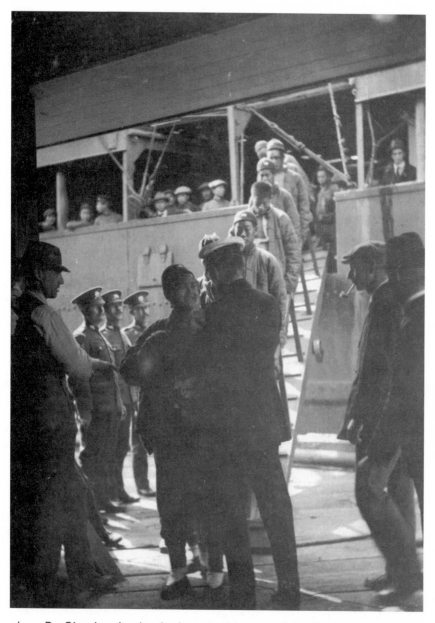

above Dr. Glendenning beginning a head count of detainees, 1917.
METCHOSIN SCHOOL MUSEUM

opposite This tall Mongolian member of the CLC caught the attention of one William Head school girl. METCHOSIN SCHOOL MUSEUM

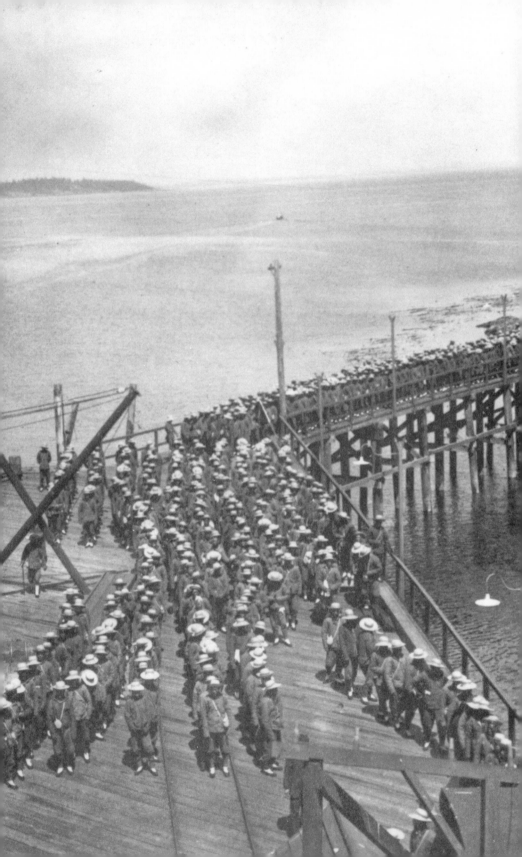

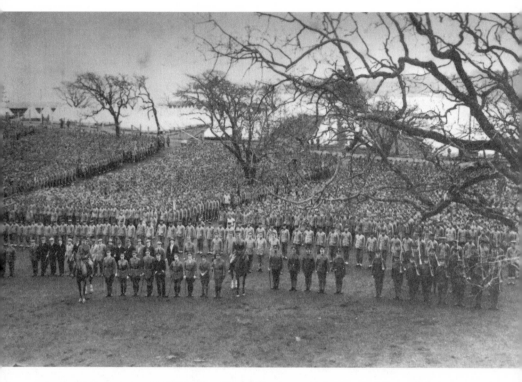

above CLC members at William Head Station getting a preview of the military discipline they would encounter in France.
METCHOSIN SCHOOL MUSEUM

opposite Ready to proceed from the wharf to their encampment, the CLC volunteers had little to look forward to at William Head.
METCHOSIN SCHOOL MUSEUM

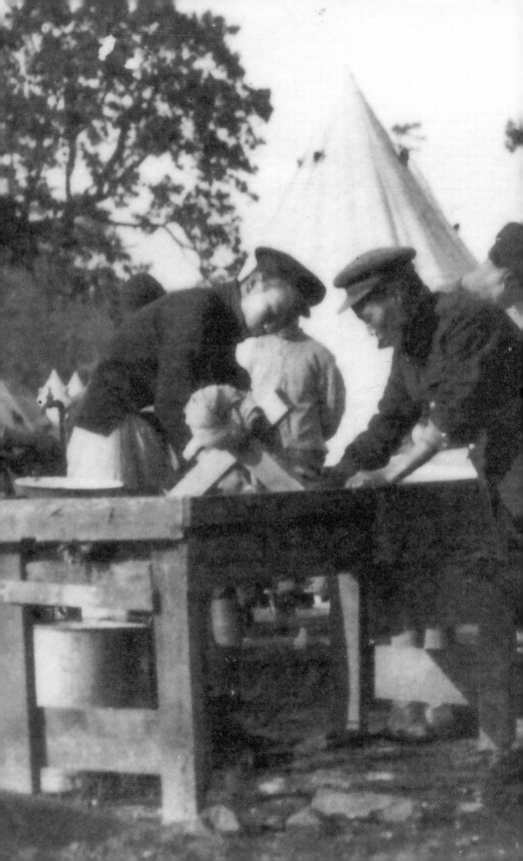

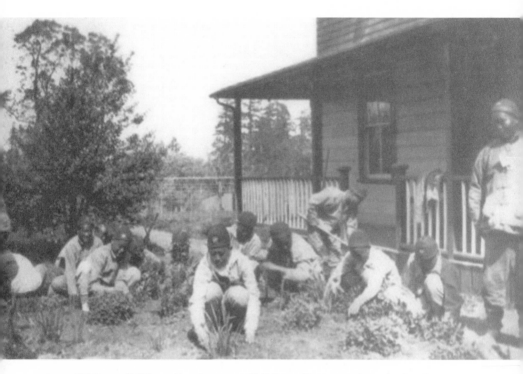

above While at William Head, many CLC battalion members helped with the upkeep of the grounds. METCHOSIN SCHOOL MUSEUM

opposite A work gang doing laundry for their CLC battalion while at William Head. Note the bell tent in the background.
METCHOSIN SCHOOL MUSEUM

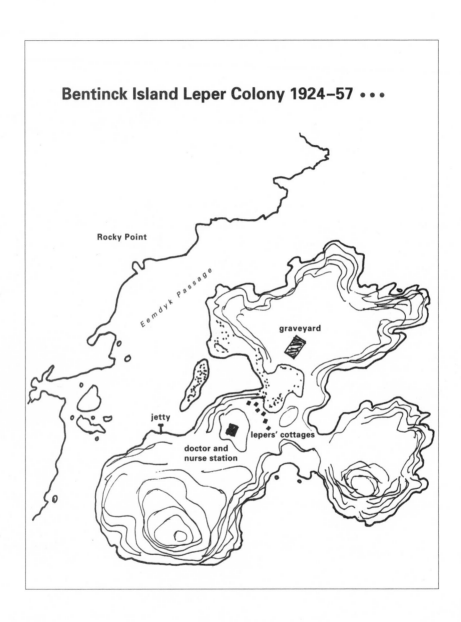

Bentinck Island Leper Colony 1924–57 • • •

Rocky Point

Eemdyk Passage

graveyard

jetty

lepers' cottages

doctor and
nurse station

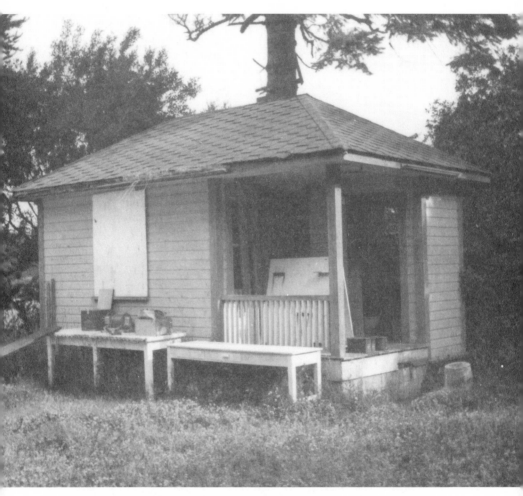

This leper's cabin on Bentinck Island was humble, but it was a vast improvement from the facilities on D'Arcy Island some fifty years before.

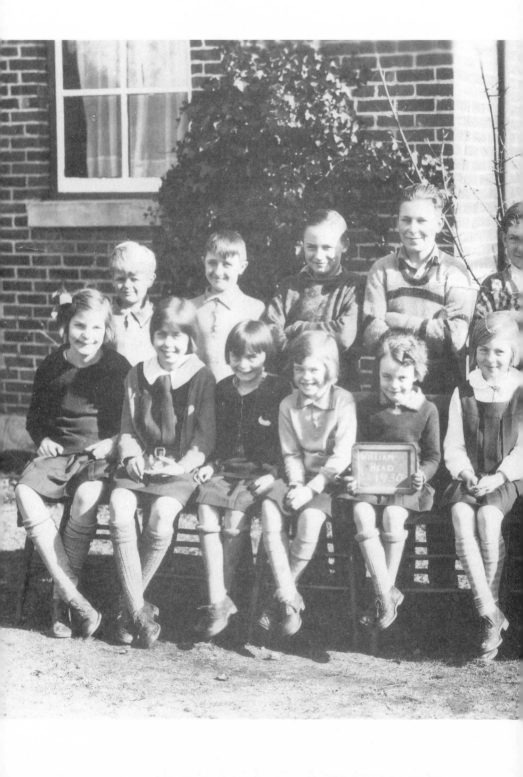

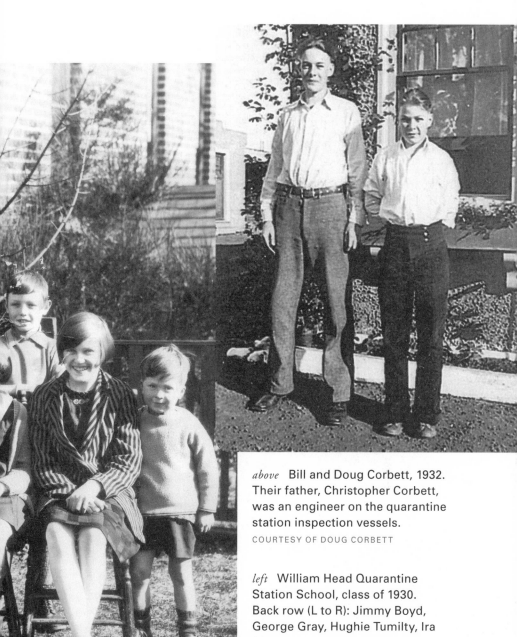

above Bill and Doug Corbett, 1932.
Their father, Christopher Corbett,
was an engineer on the quarantine
station inspection vessels.

COURTESY OF DOUG CORBETT

left William Head Quarantine
Station School, class of 1930.
Back row (L to R): Jimmy Boyd,
George Gray, Hughie Tumilty, Ira
Brown, Ian Gibson. Front row
(L to R): Dorothy Shrewsbury, Joan
Hawkins, Allison Shrewsbury,
Joceyln Lee, Betty Shrewsbury,
Faith Lee, Hazel Hawkins,
Mary Gray, Mike Lee.

COURTESY OF FAITH WALTON (NÉE LEE)

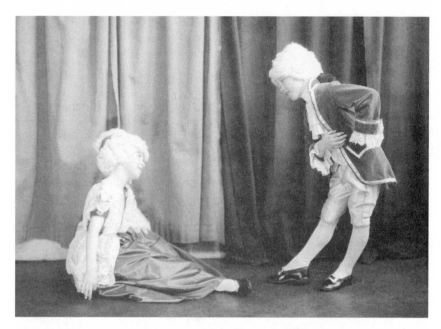

above Faith Lee and Ian Gibson performing at the station school's Christmas concert in 1933. Gibson went on to become an internationally acclaimed ballet dancer. COURTESY OF FAITH WALTON (NÉE LEE)

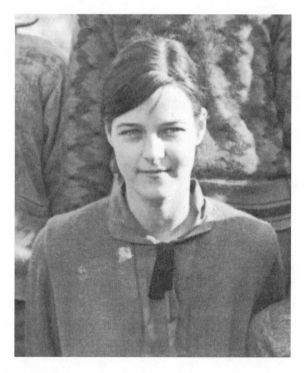

left Noni Bolton at sixteen in 1938. She would later become an intelligence officer in Britain's overseas operations and dated a few of the "spitfire" pilots of the Battle of Britain. METCHOSIN SCHOOL MUSEUM

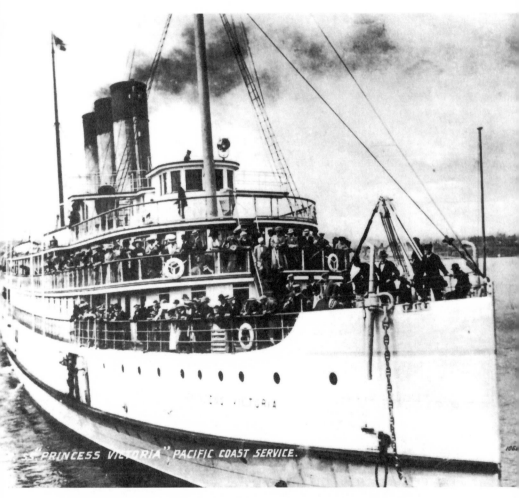

"PRINCESS VICTORIA" PACIFIC COAST SERVICE.

Replacing the *Islander*, *Princess Victoria* often carried immigrants and tourists from Victoria to Seattle and Vancouver throughout the 1910s.
METCHOSIN SCHOOL MUSEUM

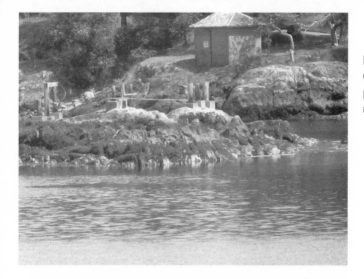

Dangerous
Chemicals Building,
present day.
PETER JOHNSON

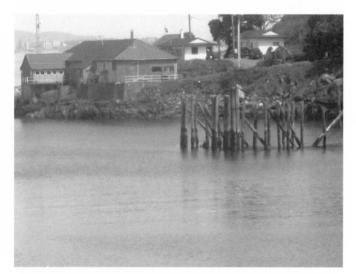

Quarantine
buildings along
the wharf and
remains of the pier,
present day.
PETER JOHNSON

Quarantine chapel
and school,
present day.
PETER JOHNSON

First-Class
Bathhouse,
present day.
PETER JOHNSON

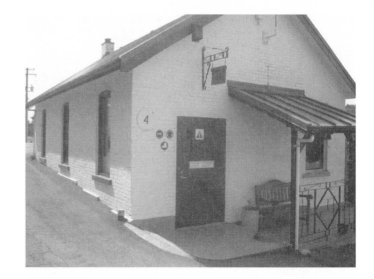

Rear of
Fumigation
Building,
present day.
PETER JOHNSON

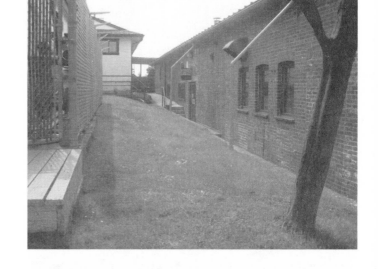

Headstone for
Julian Lucas,
quarantined from
the *Empress of
Russia*. Died at
William Head.
PETER JOHNSON

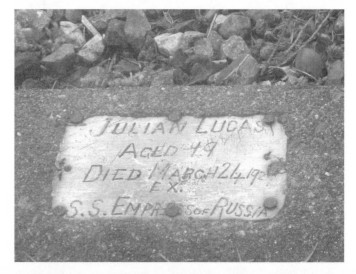

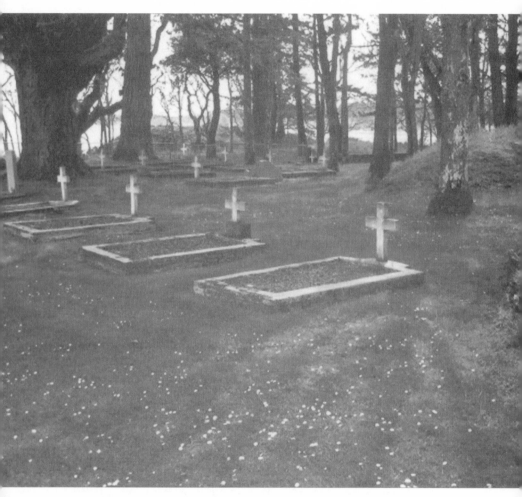

Quarantine Station Cemetery, present day. PETER JOHNSON

CHAPTER 9 // "FREE AS LARKS": THE CHILDREN OF WILLIAM HEAD

Pancake Tuesday is a very happy day,
If you don't give us a holiday, we'll all run away.

—A schoolyard chant about Shrove Tuesday, the day before the beginning of Lent[1]

When John McMullan applied for the position of teacher at the William Head Quarantine Station School on August 9, 1910, he thought he had it in the bag. He had a degree, had taught for eight years, had been a principal, and held certificates for British Columbia and Quebec. For the elementary school position to which he applied, John McMullan was dramatically overqualified. His application, however, unravelled as soon as his real motives became known. The poor man was so fed up with the horror of prairie cold that he literally begged for asylum. "I have found the winter [near Edmonton] very severe and desire to see British Columbia with the view of making it my home," he wrote in his application.[2] As impeccable as his qualifications were, John McMullan would have to find another way to make it to Lotus Land. His candidness did not cut any ice with Dr. Watt.

By 1900, the William Head Quarantine Station employed over twenty full-time staff, and many had arrived with wives and families. As positions were permanent and included such perks as on-site housing, it wasn't long before more babies bloomed like weeds. Sending the school-aged children daily through the cougar-infested woods to the one-room schoolhouse in Metchosin was out of the question, so in 1907, station chief Dr. Watt pursued federal money for an on-site school. In 1909, Ottawa responded with funding for a teacher, and a small one-storey cabin located near the staff houses was turned into a school just in time for the fall term.

Lenora Lermayne had only just immigrated to Victoria and had been a teacher in London. She was twenty-two and looking for something different from the spinsterhood that would have defined her life in Britain. Reluctantly, through Dr. Watt's urgings, Lenora agreed to accept the position, but only until the end of June 1910. She was paid $400 for the school year.

To replace her and to entice new candidates, the station school increased the annual teaching salary to $650, a whopping pay hike of 60 percent. There were several applications, though many, like John McMullan's, were put aside. Two hopeful candidates, Reta Huston and Nellie Robertson, had just finished high school (grade 11), and junior matriculation in those days was enough to qualify as an elementary school teacher in British Columbia. However, as neither had ever taught, neither had any experience of managing a group of rambunctious children, and both were only 16, their applications were discarded.

Eileen Mulcahy was well known at Victoria High School as a cultured and clever young lady. She passed the 1909 Junior Matriculation Examination with distinction and excelled in the 1910 McGill Matriculation Examination (grade 12), winning the school's Governor General's Medal. After teaching in Victoria for one year, she applied for the position at the William Head School but was rejected upon the receipt of her letter of reference from Edward Paul, Victoria's superintendent of schools. He noted, among other things that, "Miss Mulcahy has considerable force of character" and was most "efficient."[3] To Dr. Watt, that polite obfuscation intimated that she was inflexible and demanding.

* In the end, the job went to Mrs. McKenzie, a middle-aged, kindly, experienced teacher who gained the affection of the sixteen children in her class and their anxious parents. She remained at the quarantine station school until the outbreak of the First World War.

In 1915, the school was relocated to the new recreation hall. It was built for the benefit of station workers, and soon became the focus of many family activities. The hall was large enough to provide an upstairs apartment for the new live-in teacher, the energetic Miss E. Jones, while the main floor became a huge single classroom where grades one through six were taught together. On Sundays, the hall became the chapel.

It was the children who became the real ambassadors of the William Head Quarantine Station from 1920 to 1950. In their boisterous and unsophisticated energy, they roamed together freely over the nearby hills of Metchosin, and beyond toward the city of Victoria. They came to know those scattered villages, connected with everyone, and missed nothing in their probing curiosity. Their games, lore, and secret places passed as naturally between them as the skipping-rope rhymes they chanted and the codes they shared.

It was the children who ignored the sacrosanct social hierarchy that prevailed among the staff at William Head. Where medical officers only befriended administrators, groundskeepers communicated only with guards, and fumigation technicians mingled only with those who ran the boats, the children interacted with everyone. They alone came to know all the important families who lived on or off the station and also knew the poor families and their children who lived on the surrounding farms. They demanded of everyone they encountered a community-mindedness that gave the quarantine station an undeniably positive force in the life of greater Victoria.

Theirs was a thriving, unselfconscious culture, belonging to the greatest of all tribes, the worldwide fraternity of childhood. As they grew they came to understand the station's isolation and the immensity of the surrounding sea and forest, and it gave them boundless opportunities to learn self-reliance. They took those lessons and that energy into the large communities in which they would soon serve.

During the Depression and through the Second World War, it was the children of William Head who moderated the fear in the surrounding communities that the quarantine station was an edifice that stood only for sickness and death. They possessed a vitality that simply could not be ignored. In all, theirs was a divine wind. As Joan Watkins, Metchosin pioneer and childhood friend of many of the station's children, said at the age of ninety-four, "we had a rich and memorable time . . . we were as free as larks."[4]

FRANK RHODE WAS HIRED in 1915 to become the caretaker at the leper colony on D'Arcy Island. However, when officials discovered that Frank and wife, Daisy, had infant children, they realized that such a move would generate a surfeit of bad press—something that the station did not need. Instead, Frank was offered a job on the station, and his children, Christopher and Violet, began school on the site.

Little Violet Rhode was at school in 1921, and later remembered vividly how "the bathroom and washing facilities for the school children was only accessible from outside the hall."[5] Her younger brother, Christopher, was for a time the only little boy in the class, and was spoiled by everyone. But such adoration was not always the case. In the mid-1920s, Violet remembered a male teacher who was feared and unpopular with the children in Grade 5. She recalled that on several occasions one of the station's many cats would find its way into the schoolroom to be doted on by every girl in class. "On one particular day, the teacher flew into a rage, picked up the cat, swung it around his head and flung it out of the window."[6] Needless to say, the children were horrified. That teacher remained only one year.

Most teachers loved working at the William Head Station School and stayed for several years. Mrs. McKenzie taught there for four years and was succeeded by Miss Jones, Miss Winhall, the short-term "feline-flyer," and Miss Blankenbar, who remained until the beginning of the Depression. Then, like a bombshell, the dreaded Mrs. Soule arrived. She remained so long that she even struck terror into the hearts of Christopher Rhode's two daughters when they, too, attended the school some fifteen years later.

"Sergeant Major" Soule was the consummate battleaxe and ran the William Head Station School with all the authority of a field marshal. She was grey-haired and authoritarian when Mike and Faith Lee and Douglas Corbett arrived in 1931. By then her reputation had become legendary. The children found out soon enough that it was too risky to look up from their books or pass notes to one another in class. Breaking the rules was met with the punishment of standing on a chair facing the rest of the class, and some found themselves in this position on a regular basis. According to Mike Lee, whenever the boys met Mrs. Soule on the streets of the station or in Victoria, they were to stop, stand at attention, and offer her a crisp salute. She was determined to reform the young hellions if it killed her, and it nearly did.

Mrs. Soule's no-nonsense approach to child-rearing was more than the educational philosophy of the day; it was grounded in the regrets and misfortunes of her own married life. On weekends, in the early years, Mrs. Soule went home to her husband and son, Rupert, who lived off the station at nearby Rocky Point. But her husband was years older than she, and by the early 1930s he had become a feeble old man. Rupert was a drifter who had quit school early, had married young, became a logger, and drank. Mrs. Soule believed that the boys at the station school could avoid a similar future through courtesy, discipline, and hard work—which explains why they bore the brunt of her punishments while the girls got away with lighter sentences. At eighty-five, Mike Lee remembered that Mrs. Soule "thought she ran the place."[7]

When Ned Cornwall, the station's electrician, first arrived, he promised his wife they would stay for a couple of years maximum. Ned retired from William Head thirty-five years later. Their children, Molly, Betty, Brook, and Barbara, all attended the station school. They grew up and went to school with Christopher and Violet Rhode and chummed with the sons of Teddy Thomas, the station's carpenter and coffin maker. Margaret Robertson, daughter of Captain Robertson of the tender *Madge,* attended the school, and would later write articles recording their childhood adventures for the *Colonist.* Gwen, Annie, Margaret, and Hugh Tumilty, whose father was the station's chief engineer, all played with Raymond, Harold, Gerald, and Mary Gray. Percy Gray was the station's accountant and chief steward.

Beryl Nelson, daughter of Dr. Nelson (chief medical officer 1913–23), often joined in with the other children's games, though horses were her passion. The expansive, scenic grasslands and open trails of the station gave Beryl room to ride in safety. Often she rode with Dr. Tremayne's two children. Together, they all ran with Faith, Jocelyn, Geoffrey, and Mike Lee, children of the station's groundskeeper, and with Hazel and Joan Hawkins, children of a station gardener who had grown up in Metchosin.

Betty and Dorothy Shrewsbury were the children of Bill Shrewsbury, a customs officer stationed at William Head during the late 1930s. They roamed with Ian Gibson, the acrobatic son of James Gibson, one of the guards. Dr. Boyd's young son, Jimmy, often explored the edge of the sea with Billy and Douglas Corbett, whose father captained one of the station's quarantine tenders.

In the mid-1930s, Mavis and Stanley Bain, children of chief medical officer Dr. Bain (1936–39), attended the station school. Ira Brown and his sister, the children of Dr. Chester Brown, the station's chief medical officer from 1923 to 1934, went to the school as well. Both were scholars and readily passed the entrance exams necessary to attend high school in Victoria.

While the public school system in Victoria was a provincial responsibility, the federal government assumed responsibility for the school at William Head, and consequently its curriculum was continually scrutinized to ensure it met the requirements for high school entrance. As Douglas Corbett remembered, "the provincial inspector would come out and grill us on the subjects we could expect on the exams. He was supposed to come unannounced, but somehow Jocelyn Lee's mother always heard of his imminent arrival and conveniently . . . kept her children home 'sick' on the days of his visit." It turned out, however, that the inspector was a friendly fellow and Jocelyn was smart. She wrote, "he helped me with all the answers, and so I got the top marks on the exams."[8]

Barbara and Robert Cox were the children of Dr. Cox, assistant medical officer at the station with Dr. Brown in the early 1930s. Being older than the others, they befriended the two Robinson boys who lived off the station at Rocky Point. Mr. Robinson was disabled and had no means of getting his children into the village school in Metchosin, so they were allowed to attend classes at William Head, as were Peter and Desmond Bradford, also of Rocky Point.

Many of the children were given piano lessons in the early 1930s by Mrs. MacMinn, wife of the station's customs officer. The MacMinns had immigrated to Victoria from South Africa, and Earnest had fought in the Boer War before coming to Canada to become a customs official in Port Alberni. Their five children, Richard, Albert, Jesse, Flo, and Earnest, swelled the school's numbers to over twenty-five.

When the Second World War began, young Ira Brown joined the Canadian army and served in the Italian campaign in 1943. Fighting to secure the "toe" of Italy for the Allied landing, Ira became ill in the rugged, rock-strewn hills south of Mount Etna. He was one of the lucky ones who survived the campaign, but was hospitalized with severe amoebic dysentery. His friend and station school classmate Frank Rhode enlisted as soon as he reached seventeen. Eager to participate in the great adventure, his friends Desmond Bradford and Geoffrey Lee followed Frank to the front. Desmond and Geoffrey never made it home. Desmond was killed in action near Berlin in the latter stages of the war, and Geoffrey, who had become a Royal Canadian Air Force observer, was shot down over Cologne.

Violet Rhode remembered another wartime incident that shaped the quarantine station years before. In 1917, as the First World War dragged on, Violet, seven and at school, saw thousands of Chinese arrive at William Head. They were part of the CLC en route to the trenches of northern France. Violet saw them on two separate occasions. "The Station's landscape was covered with white bell tents with huge caldrons set up for cooking. I can remember a Chinese man that stood out, or should I say, stood above the rest of his countrymen. He was well over six feet tall. He went off to war one day, dressed in his pale blue-grey uniform of baggy pants, front button jacket and little round hat"[9]

Two years would pass before the CLC was repatriated to China and en route home they were again processed through the William Head Quarantine Station. Violet Rhode was still at school when they returned. "We watched and watched as they began to return home and once again pass through the station, dressed in the strangest outfits consisting of German helmets, and bits and scraps of Allied clothing . . . then one day, still towering above all the rest . . . there he was, home safe, and sound."[10]

By the mid-1930s, the enrolment at the station school was large enough for it to hold dramatic presentations for the whole William Head community. The school choir sang at the Harvest Festival, while on November 5, the youngest helped their fathers gather wood for the evening burning of Guy Fawkes, a custom that had not yet been eclipsed by the practice of Halloween.

The highlight of the year was the school's Christmas concert. It was an important community affair and preparation began early each fall. Parents made period costumes, in which Ian Gibson and Faith Lee, being similar in size, would dance a seventeenth-century minuet, and Betty Shrewsbury and Jimmy Boyd would perform a German "Clog Dance." Others performed in the slick revue known as "Mrs. Jarley's Wax Works" in which several children adopted the guise of wind-up dolls and danced in unison until their "springs" ran down. Others recited Stanley Holloway verses or performed Scottish folk dances in authentic kilts and breeches. The William Head Station's orchestra, which several of the older children belonged to, provided the music.[11]

• The recreation hall became the venue for this annual Christmas gala, which was eagerly attended by family and friends of station workers from all the surrounding communities. From these beginnings, the light-footed Ian Gibson would grow up to train as a ballet dancer, first in Vancouver and then in France. During the mid-1930s, he danced throughout Europe with the company of Anna Pavlova of the famous Ballets Russes. When it played in New York just before the outbreak of the Second World War, Ian became an instant star. When the war began, Ian joined the fledgling Submarine Service of the Royal Canadian Navy. He survived, but just barely. After the war, Ian Gibson simply disappeared from the world of dance, perhaps disillusioned or afraid that he had lost his technique.[12] He eventually became an executive in a taxi company in Alpine, New Jersey, but would never dance or resurface at William Head again.

On most Sundays during the 1920s, Violet Rhode's father, Frank, rowed from the quarantine station across to Rocky Point to pick up the young Reverend Henry Bolton of St. Mary the Virgin, the Anglican Church in Metchosin. As part of his mission, Reverend Bolton travelled out to Rocky Point and held a Sunday service for local settlers. Then, complete with white collar, bible, fishing rod, and "floppy hat sporting the latest lures,"[13] Reverend Bolton conducted an afternoon service for the station staff. According to Violet Rhode, church services were initially held in the second-class hospital, and later in the chapel. They were followed by the interminably long Sunday school lessons for the children given by one of the mothers. During these protracted afternoons, young Reverend Bolton often disappeared; he'd gone fishin'.[14]

Arthur Lee's second son, Michael, was delivered in the station's hospital by Dr. Brown on August 6, 1925. Reverend Bolton was only too glad to christen him into the Anglican faith. He was placed in a makeshift font and "baptized with water from the kitchen kettle."[15] Hazel and Joan Hawkins were also confirmed into the Anglican faith in their mid-teens by Reverend Bolton. But Mike Lee and his friends soon tired of Reverend Bolton's moralizing; they found him "sedate, ineffectual, and boring."[16]

To say Mike Lee and Stanley Bain were hooligans would be an understatement. Mike's father worked as a groundskeeper, while Stanley was the son of Dr. Bain. Stanley's sister, Mavis, was an angel, but young Stanley was a boy with attitude. As youngsters, Mike Lee and Stanley Bain had the run of the place, and when they got together, they got into trouble. Passenger traffic had almost ceased completely at the William Head Quarantine Station from the late 1930s until the end of war, and it was during this time that many of the older detention buildings at the station fell into disrepair. Mike and Stanley, now on the edge of puberty, were caught on one occasion breaking the windows of several of these abandoned buildings. Mrs. Soule forced Stanley to make a public apology before everyone on the station, while his administrative father stood by, humiliated. Mike's father gave his wayward son a sound whipping. Mrs. Soule, cracker-jack battleaxe that she was, knew more about family life and class distinctions at the station than she was publicly prepared to say.

There is no question that Mike Lee and Stanley Bain knew about the smuggling that went on at the William Head Quarantine Station during the early 1930s. Part of the contract that allowed for a Canada Customs Officer to be placed at William Head was the condition that station personnel would assist customs officers in patrolling the coast. The enemy was prohibition. Most of the American east coast had declared the sale and manufacture of intoxicating liquor illegal in 1915. When Washington and eighteen other states outlawed the consumption of booze that same year, the market soared for imported liquor and homemade moonshine, especially from British Columbia.

Canada had introduced prohibition in 1917, but in British Columbia, public demonstrations throughout 1920 forced a plebiscite to repeal the legislation and for thirteen glorious years, until 1933 when America, too, repealed the law, British Columbia enjoyed a thriving rum-running subculture. Contraband booze was regularly carried from countless coves along the British Columbia coast across the Juan de Fuca Strait to similar havens near Port Angeles or Port Townsend in Washington State. The William Head Quarantine Station became the perfect location for several of these ventures.

Faith Lee remembered seeing the smugglers directly. When the Lees first moved to William Head, the family lived in a cottage overlooking the rocks at the very seaward end of the peninsula. One of Arthur Lee's jobs was to act as nightwatchman over quarantined Asian immigrants who were detained in the nearby Chinese House. Faith proudly proclaimed, "Father was never afraid of anything, often climbing over the foreshore bedrock in the inky blackness to the seashore to catch Asian escapees or watch for the rum-runners in their dark, slick craft."[17]

Faith remembered being worried one night as she watched her father head for the promontory. An instant later, "she saw several men run through the station grounds toward the wharf carrying wooden cases which were dropped into a waiting boat."[18]

In 1932, when Doug Corbett was in grade five, he often saw his father and customs officers board the quarantine boat *Salucan V* to make the run from William Head west to Sooke looking for Johnny Schnarr's infamous, high-powered rum-running launch *Kitnayakwa*. Doug also saw the fast, American-registered police cutter *Adversis* and the Canadian *Imperator* at the station's wharf. Though most of these patrols came to naught, the existence of smuggling from the William Head Quarantine Station remained a closely held secret among the children until after the war.

Queen Victoria's birthday was always a red-letter day in the life of the quarantine station children. In the days before the all-weather road into Victoria was built, as many families as possible boarded the *Madge* for the annual, often unpleasant voyage into the city to participate in the mid-May celebrations. The *Madge* was difficult to manoeuvre in heavy seas, and once clear of the headlands of Parry Bay, she would inevitably begin her unnerving roll. Violet Rhode remembered being seasick many times while wearing her finest white spring dress, but it never deterred her or any of her young friends. The David Spencer float in the Inner Harbour was always reserved for the William Head boat on the Victoria Day weekend.

The schoolgirls of both communities readily found each other and together they watched the parade along Government Street, chatted incessantly over ices, and promenaded in all their white finery in front of the Empress Hotel.

"Did you know that a few years ago Edward, Prince of Wales, danced until dawn in the Empress's Crystal Ballroom with so-and-so's older sister?" one of them would sputter, giggling to the others. The boys ran from all this nonsense into the vastness of Beacon Hill Park, but the promise of food and treasure hunts and the sound of bandstand music wafting redolently over the low hills, brought them back. During the Depression, those at the quarantine station had permanent employment and money to spend. For hard-pressed Victoria shopkeepers, the arrival of station families was a godsend.

Quarantine was the business of the William Head Station, so ship stories abounded in the lore of the children. The fear of smallpox required that the children on-site were to be vaccinated every two years. Many, like Faith Lee and her friends, tried to hide on vaccination day, often in the folds of backyard tents. Older brothers gleefully reported them to those with the dreaded needle. As the red sores of vaccinations healed, stories of inbound ocean ships halted by quarantine at William Head became endlessly fascinating.

Violet Rhode recalled seeing the famous passenger liner *Monteagle* waiting for clearance in Parry Bay. The *Monteagle* had gained fame through its daring rescue of sixty-six of the seventy crew members of the sinking French freighter *Hsin Tien* in the China Sea in 1921. She also saw the American mail liner *President Jefferson* when it docked at the station on September 16, 1923, bringing with it the first 468 refugees from a catastrophic earthquake in Japan. They were given emergency accommodation at the quarantine station, and Violet was witness to all the goings-on.

With over 100,000 dead, Tokyo, Yokohama, and Yokosuka were virtually destroyed by the quake. When the *President Jefferson* arrived at the station, Violet recalled, "the entire international press was on hand [and] in a mad scramble to get the first eye-witness reports. Three seaplanes had been hired to rush pictures to the United States. One crashed on landing, probably gaining the dubious distinction of the first seaplane crash on the coast. One newsman aboard a speedboat was reported to have $10,000 to offer passengers who had exclusive pictures of the Japanese disaster."[19] Because cholera had broken out on the *President Jefferson* as a consequence of the quake, the ship had been quarantined and no one, including the station's children, was allowed anywhere near the quay.

* One epic tale of ships and the sea eclipsed all the others in Violet Rhode's youth at the station. On October 13, 1929, the *Empress of Canada* was inbound from New York and San Francisco. A band of white fog curtained the Juan de Fuca Strait and completely obscured the Canadian shore. Coastal pilot Captain George Roberts was in charge as the ship slowly made its way around Race Rocks toward the William Head Quarantine Station for clearance. The official record stated that the *Empress of Canada* had "strayed off course," and was farther north than its presumed position. Though moving dead slow through the morning gloom, the *Empress of Canada* suddenly struck the promontory of Albert Head. Its 21,000-ton momentum shoved its bows over one hundred feet up onto the jagged rocks of the infamous peninsula. Its double bottom was punctured by stone pinnacles and its hull was held, vise-like, in a sharp stone cleft. The ship was firmly grounded. Steamship and salvage officials worried that if a southeast gale blew in, the famous liner would be wrecked. But it didn't happen. Fortunately, the fog lifted, the weather remained calm, and crowds of curious onlookers from Victoria and William Head gathered to watch the salvage operation of the pride of the *Empress* fleet. It took some careful blasting of the rock pinnacles, seven tugs, and two days to pull the *Empress of Canada* free.

The old fog signal fixed at the very end of the William Head Peninsula might have been partly to blame and the children knew it. It was little more than a water-powered bell, and a long pipe carried water to it from the station. The water turned a wheel, which activated a striker that regularly boomed the bell's monotone horn across the fog-ridden waters of Parry Bay. The trouble was, the pipe had a dip in it, and in winter when the water failed to drain, it froze and split the pipe. The children reported the incident, and the bell was replaced with a more powerful propane horn. On this day, however, even the new system wasn't enough.

By 1912, Dr. Watt had range lights and a sea buoy fixed off William Head and their positions marked on hydrographic charts. Ships requiring clearance from the quarantine station swung wide around the lighthouse and currents at Race Rocks, keeping a watchful eye out for the range lights and the sea buoy. Yet even these new measures failed the *Empress of Canada*.

As the taffrail log clicked off the distance run and vector lines drawn on charts accounted for tide and currents, an alert pilot should have been able to steer his ship safely toward the station wharf. But the official off-course version of the grounding of the *Empress of Canada* differed from what the children overheard. Diana Jenkins, daughter of Dr. Roy Bertram Jenkins, chief medical officer at William Head from 1939 to 1957, recounted the dramatic tale.

As per the record, Diana knew that medical officers along with customs and immigration officials boarded the ship while it was still out in the strait. But Diana's story contained an element sacred to all teenage girls, a reference to young love. That morning, on the bridge of the *Empress of Canada*, the officer of the watch had just received a letter from his beloved in England. Whether it was an acceptance of a proposal or a rejection, Diana was unsure, but the officer was so intent on its contents that he failed to order the ship's telegraph back from its "Dead Slow Ahead" position and the ship ghosted its way through the fog of Parry Bay and ran onto the rocks of Albert Head.[20] Beth Harmon was nine at the time, and she later remembered seeing the huge liner firmly embedded on the peninsula all the way to the first of its three huge funnels. As a result of the accident, the Canadian government installed a lighthouse and foghorn at Albert Head.[21]

Beth and her schoolmates grew up hearing the distinctive winter wails of the foghorns on the headlands near the quarantine station. The muted, doleful cry of the horn on the end of the Albert Head Peninsula they named "Mournful Maud," while the blatant trumpet of the horn at Race Rocks became known as "Billowing Billy."[22]

During the war, the famous Cunard liner *Queen Mary* was comman-
deered by the British Army and converted into a troop ship. In 1944, it was
often seen by the children inbound to William Head carrying thousands of
wounded soldiers home from the Pacific theatre of the war. The *Queen Mary*
was ideal for this task, not only because it was spacious but because it held,
for fourteen years, the Blue Riband, speeding across the seas faster than any
other ship afloat. Diana Jenkins delighted in telling one tale about the ship
because her mother, Evelyn (known as Eve), was central to it.

Eve's husband, chief medical officer Dr. Jenkins, was out on a station boat inspecting another inbound ship requiring quarantine clearance.
When the station phone rang in the superintendent's office, Eve picked up
the receiver. A voice asked, "When is the *Queen Mary* arriving?"

Realizing that such information was classified, Mrs. Jenkins replied that
in order to get such information, the gentleman should call "Mary Hill."

"Who in the hell is Mary Hill?" the man replied.

"If you don't know who Mary Hill is, then you are not qualified to
know the time of the *Queen Mary*'s arrival!" Eve was nervous but firm.
She hung up, having possibly disgruntled a correspondent from Toronto,
or, more seriously, uncovered an Axis agent. The man's comment belied
his motives in that "Mary Hill" was the name of the 5th British Columbia
Coast Brigade's coastal defence battery located on the high bluff (Mary
Hill), near the William Head Quarantine Station. Had he been a legitimate
reporter or lived in the area, he would have readily known such information.
Diana and her childhood friends believed her mother had probably saved
many lives.[23]

In 1930, Beth Ellwood was ten, old enough to help her father run his
general store in Metchosin. The store was contracted to supply groceries
and dry goods to the William Head Quarantine Station through to the
end of the Second World War. During the 1930s, Beth often travelled with
her father to the station, where she befriended several children her own
age. That association became critical when the threat of infectious diseases
loomed. When a ship was placed under quarantine, especially with cases
of smallpox on board, the children of the station were particularly vulnerable. On such occasions they were evacuated from William Head to stay

with various families in Metchosin and the surrounding communities. The Ellwood family home was not large, and even Beth's three sisters, Valerie, Enid, and Gwennie-May shared bedrooms. Suddenly, for weeks in April 1927, the Ellwood home resounded to the squeals of five more delighted station children.[24]

Joan Pears recalled being taken around by her "Uncle Guy" Pears, medic and caretaker for the Bentinck Island Leper Colony, with her young quarantine station friends in one of the station's large, old longboats, waving to the lepers and the Native fishermen off Rocky Point. Joan admitted reluctantly to landing more than once at the leper colony and engaging in a linguistic pantomime with the congenial lepers. She knew it was a dangerous thing to do, and if she were found out, she would have been punished. Her sister Beryl worked in the Ellwood General Store in Metchosin, so if Joan had become contagious, the results might have been catastrophic.

During his late adolescence, Mike Lee often "stood in" for the Bentinck Island nurse when it was necessary for her to travel to Victoria to replenish the colony's supplies. Mike, too, did not hesitate to associate with the lepers, and he became especially friendly with one Japanese leper who was particularly adept with tools. The leper's resolve to survive his affliction and become a carpenter had a great influence on young Mike Lee and he, along with Mrs. Soule, steered the boy away from further adolescent deviance.

Besides the nearby leper colony, there were other places at the quarantine station that were strictly off limits for the children. A hut located near the fumigation building was full of dangerous chemicals and, supposedly, kept under lock and key. However, Joan and Hazel Hawkins, along with Faith Lee, often needed "cakes" to complete their childhood game of playing house. The cakes of yellow sulphur, kept in the hut, were the perfect size and shape. How the girls managed to secure these round and yellow "desserts" and "feed" them to their dolls along with "high tea" no one ever said.

As at Race Rocks, the currents around Bentinck Island were always fierce. Doug Corbett remembered seeing killer whales only feet from the shore as they gathered at the northern end of Eemdyk Passage, waiting for salmon. Often, even the whales were sucked through the passage into Pedder Bay. In 1930, several Aboriginal fishermen were drowned there when they slipped off the rocks into the raging tidal flow. It was there, too, that Doug Corbett saw a huge North Pacific octopus entangled around a log shoot through the rapids out to sea. Despite the danger, the children of the William Head Station continued to venture down to the shore to play or buy salmon from Natives who, set up their fishing camp beside the raging waters in October.

In the 1920s, the William Head Quarantine Station was remote from Victoria. That was a boon to its mandate, but its isolation posed some dangers for the children. Where first-growth wilderness touched the arbutus groves of the peninsula, there were cougars. At ten years old, Marjorie Rhode saw the family dog cornered by a cougar beneath the back steps of her home. It took two station workers, Jim Rainy and Captain Cole, using all their strength to pull the dog from the grip of the cougar's jaws. The bleeding dog was frantic, and Marjorie, full of tears, drew near. Undeterred, the cougar eyed new prey. Seconds before it pounced on the little girl, Jim Rainy shot the beast. He sold it to a restaurant in Chinatown for twenty dollars.

The William Head Peninsula is a rocky twenty-metre-high, sloping headland with an occasional ravine cutting down to the sea. During the winter, cold and snow were not uncommon. The boys at the station and their friends from Metchosin often built a long toboggan run from the laboratory down to the ocean shore at "School Beach." They would keep the run open through the slush until the end of March.

The huge sweep of Parry Bay north to Albert Head became the summer playground for the children of Metchosin and the station. In the lee of the cold winds from the Juan de Fuca Strait, Parry Bay was itself divided into three separate haunts. At Taylor Beach, the water was too cold for swimming, though because of its huge log deposits, it was a great place to built huts and forts. Weir's Beach, the locale for the station school's annual picnic, was often windy, but its small tidal pools were full of fascinating creatures. Witty's Beach, near the lagoon, was "just right" for a lazy afternoon swim.

Of them all, Taylor Beach was the most enduring because, as the children of the school matured into teenagers, the logs at Taylor Beach proved not only great for rafts but also for other, more nefarious and carnal pleasures. During the war, when the girls of the school had reached their teens, some ventured out on dates with the teenage boys from the surrounding communities. All knew of a special hut near Taylor Beach, and more than likely had contributed to its upkeep. The logs of Taylor Beach served their hormones well, and the cramped and hidden retreat emboldened many an only-too-willing young lad and his inquisitive lassie to use the place to engage in some heavy breathing. The Taylor Beach hut in those glorious Arcadian days was redolent with perfume and the memory of many an undone button.

The adolescent boys on the station were like spies, alert to the movement of all girls in the area. As Mike Lee recounted, "If any family settled on any of the surrounding farms, it didn't take long for us to check out the girls."[25] After the war, when he was in his early twenties, Mike Lee found work on a farm in East Sooke. When he learned that a new family had moved into the nearby Rocky Point community, he cruised by in his new Ford coupe. Mike discovered that the Thornette family had a teenage daughter named Elsi. Mike married her in 1948, and in 1950, joined the quarantine service and worked at the William Head Quarantine Station as a deckhand on the *Salucan*. He remained at the station until it closed.

In July 1923, a young adventurer from Metchosin went voyaging on a raft built from Taylor Beach logs only to find himself caught in the strong tidal current that swept around the southern tip of Vancouver Island. Horrified, his young friends saw their pal disappear "halfway to Port Angeles," becoming little more than a dark speck on the scattered, white waves of the Juan de Fuca Strait. One of the children ran to Beth Ellwood's mother at the nearby general store in Metchosin. Frantic, Bee Ellwood called Dr. Chester Brown at the quarantine station, and in an instant he was on the *Madge* and out into the formidable seas. Near sunset, Dr. Brown found the young lad, hypothermic and just barely clinging to his raft. That episode made Chester Brown a hero in the settlement.

Though it was strictly against Ottawa's policy, Dr. Brown often slipped away from William Head during his tenure as chief medical officer to attend to the cuts, scrapes, and bruises of the children who lived in the nearby communities. Every day for three weeks during the summer of 1925, as part of his new-found "family practice," Dr. Brown travelled to Metchosin to change the dressing on Beth Ellwood's severely burned foot when she accidentally stepped into a campfire at Witty's Beach. Dr. Brown became the only physician the children allowed to do their required vaccinations as it was said that his needles for smallpox and other infectious diseases never hurt. Chester, as he became known among them, was adored.

As dangerous and attractive as the beaches around William Head were, there was one other area even more beguiling to the girls who lived on the station: the military barracks located at the end of Pedder Bay. (Pearson College of the Pacific now occupies that location.) In 1940, hundreds of young soldiers from across Canada paraded about the grounds, and though the military camp was guarded and isolated, many of the young men in uniform were spied upon by the girls and often seen in nearby Colwood and Metchosin.

Bookish and reserved at seventeen, demure Faith Lee had a huge crush on one soldier. Young Ivan Simmons from Victoria had joined the reserves and was stationed at Mary Hill. In 1937, Japan was at war with China and vowed to dominate all of Southeast Asia. The Allies watched Japan's every move and, as a precaution, placed a gun battery on Mary Hill. Faith fell madly in love with Ivan and the two were married in mid-1940.

When war in the Pacific exploded in 1941, Ivan went overseas and became a war photographer. Faith had become pregnant before he left, but Ivan chose to remain in France and, after two years of separation, the two divorced. Faith reclaimed her maiden name and called her only child Geoffrey in memory of her fallen older brother. Faith raised her child alone and twenty years would pass before Faith Lee would marry again.

Joan Pears lived on a farm in Metchosin and never attended the quarantine station school. But she and the Ellwood sisters, Beth, Enid, Valerie, and Gwennie-May, befriended the children at the quarantine facility. They often played tennis with them on courts reserved for first-class detainees.

Noni Bolton was the daughter of Reverend Bolton, who conducted Anglican services in the station's chapel. She and Joan Pears rode their horses together. Brook Cornwall and Ira Brown were close friends, as were Diana

Jenkins and Phyllis Houghton of Benacres Farm in Metchosin. Diana and Phyllis also rode together, often with their friend Ann Debney, who lived in Edmonton but visited during the summers. Benacres would later produce some of the finest thoroughbreds for British Columbia's racing circuit.

Elementary school life at the station sped by, and high school in Victoria with its "two whole floors of class-rooms, male teachers and boys like you never saw"[26] caused William Head parents and adolescents alike to shudder with anticipation, as Joan Watkins recalled. Victoria High was some distance from the quarantine station, so getting there in the early years proved difficult. In the 1930s, Percy Gray used to drive his own children, Mary, Gerald, Ray, and Harold, along with the two Lee girls, Faith and Jocelyn, down the winding country road into the city. When his son Gerald graduated from high school and began work at the Land Registry Office in Victoria, he drove the family car full of girls into Victoria.

Romances did develop, but dating was difficult. It was known that Gerald Gray had a huge crush on Enid Ellwood; the trouble was that Beth, Enid's younger sister, was also in love with him. On the days when Gerald drove the Lee girls and other young ladies into Victoria, the silence from the back seat was palpable. "Talk about painful," said Faith. When Enid never returned Gerald's interest, Beth Ellwood dated her beloved Gerald for a time, but the demands of work, matriculation exams, the growing uncertainty of conditions in Europe, parental vigilance, and the hardships of the Depression prevented most couples from becoming serious.

Christopher Rhode, who had just found work at the station, however, persevered. He and his high school sweetheart, Marjorie, were married in 1931. Not taking any chances, Dr. Tremayne chose to drive his two daughters into the city for school himself.

The early darkness of winter, the fierce gales, the felled trees, the poor roads, and the long daily commute soon proved too much, and Mrs. Lee, the gardener's wife at the station, rented a house for the girls in Victoria. As house mother, she took on the task of reigning in her own children, as well as the Hawkins girls and a host of other high-spirited, irrepressible female adolescents. When windfall blocked the roads, one of the station's boats would make a special run into Victoria on Monday mornings, laden with lethargic teenage girls, and meet them again Fridays, bursting now with rumours and romance.

As the Depression deepened, those parents with full-time employment at the William Head Quarantine Station were considered lucky. Their on-site housing was supplied with coal, wood, and electricity, and all upkeep and repairs were the responsibility of the federal government. Those who lived in the rural communities of Metchosin and the hills beyond suffered humiliating poverty. Joan Pears's family was dirt poor and she recalled, "I couldn't afford the textbooks for high school, so I had to go to the City Hall in Victoria and demand them. They made me pay ten cents to get them. Then, three weeks before my final matriculation exams, city officials called them in."[27] She faced exams with no texts from which to study. Joan graduated, but didn't go to her 1932 high school convocation; her parents couldn't afford the cloth to make her a dress.

• The Reverend Henry Bolton and his daughter became a fixture over the years at the William Head Quarantine Station. Nora, or "Noni" as she was called, was not, however, exactly his own. She was related to Mrs. Bolton, perhaps a niece, and was raised by the Boltons. Spirited, intelligent, and rebellious, Noni taxed the patience of her adopted parents right from the beginning. As a child, she was afraid of nothing and could be intimidating to some. Joan loved her nerve. On one occasion, as Gwennie-May and her sister Beth ventured to school on their bikes, a Clydesdale horse on the road beside them reared up and knocked Gwennie down, breaking one of her front teeth. Mr. Ellwood carried his bleeding daughter home and laid her on her bed. When her mother saw her bloodied face, she passed out. Noni witnessed the accident, went looking, and found the missing tooth. She then tried to glue it back into Gwennie's bleeding mouth. It didn't take, but it did cement a long-standing family relationship.

When Noni turned sixteen, the Reverend Bolton bought her a Model T Ford so she could drive herself to Victoria High School. She promptly careened off into a new sunrise of boys. After graduation, she and Joan, who had become best friends, were accepted into nursing. Joan's parents couldn't afford the cost of room and board at Victoria College, so, as Noni studied,

Joan remained at home in Metchosin. She tried journalism, but it did not pay well. In the midst of the Depression, and in the full flower of her youth, Joan Pears picked berries for six long years.

As they matured, Noni and Joan remained best friends and often accompanied Reverend Bolton as he ministered Anglican services throughout the Gulf Islands. For something to do, Noni and Joan began to serve tea at the many church fetes in the island settlements, and made passing acquaintances with many of the strapping young men in this pristine Eden. Within a short time, many would be called off to war and some of the best would never return.

Joan and Noni couldn't afford the area tennis club, to which the Ellwoods and many of their well-off quarantine station school gang belonged, so they simply danced to the new swing music broadcast over the radio. During this time, Noni began to find the old station gang "a bit stuffy."[28] Moreover, she had outgrown the religious constraints of her father.

From 1937 to 1938, Joan Pears attended dances in Victoria church halls, where bands such as Matt Kenney and his Western Gentlemen were broadcast over the CBC. In September 1939, Joan met George Watkins during an intermission. Though George had just joined the army, he used to hitchhike out to Metchosin to see his new girl. Immediately after their engagement, George was posted to Camp Shilo for training as a gunner. Joan followed George to Manitoba, and married him in Brandon in 1940. Just as quickly, he was sent overseas. In one heart-stopping letter home, George told his bride that his division had been selected for the invasion of Sicily.[29]

Noni Bolton never did finish nursing. As a student nurse at Royal Jubilee Hospital, she had discovered real men, and along with several of her classmates, she was expelled from Victoria College for missing too many evening curfews. Unfazed, Nonie found work and further independence as a laboratory technologist. But she was long past church fetes and Christian certitude. Some said that her conservative, anxious father packed her off to their strict Huguenot relatives in Lincolnshire, England. Some simply thought that Noni was on holidays in Britain when the Second World War began and couldn't get home. Either way, she was free. Like the Lady of Shalott, Noni demanded more of life than what was presented in the mirror-like environment of William Head.

In England, Noni joined the Women's Auxiliary Air Force (WAAF) and soon became a section officer in Fighter Operations, having access to the classified information of Britain's Fighter Command. In 1942, she married Squadron Leader Tony da Costa, a fighter pilot who had helped save Britain, flying in the glorious Spitfires during the Battle of Britain.

When the war began, the Canadian army took over the second-class hospital and detention barracks at the William Head Quarantine Station. The peninsula occupied an important strategic wartime location, commanding an overlook toward the naval base at Esquimalt and Victoria. Early in the Second World War, German pocket battleships were considered a threat in that they might steam up the Juan de Fuca Strait and shell the Esquimalt dry dock, then the largest facility on North America's west coast. After Pearl Harbor, rumour had it that Japanese submarines readily ventured up Juan de Fuca Strait, and Japanese aircraft, hugging the treetops, could swing up Haro Strait and the Gulf of Georgia to strike Vancouver with torpedoes and wing guns. It was known that Estevan Point on the west coast of Vancouver Island had been shelled by a Japanese submarine. The quarantine station at William Head was a ready target.

The Royal Canadian Navy, stationed at Esquimalt, provided the first line of defence, while a gun battery at Albert Head added longer-range fire power and anti-aircraft capability. The William Head Quarantine Station's original power plant was replaced with a more powerful forty-five-horse-power diesel-engine unit that powered its new anti-aircraft searchlights. Near the station, along the nearby beaches of the once-loved Parry Bay, Major B.D. Treatt, an expert in coastal defence, constructed a concrete pillar in the sea to mark the rise and fall of the tides in the strait, information that would be necessary if gun batteries were to accurately aim their guns at enemy ships. A small platoon of the Canadian army defended the William Head Quarantine Station and soldiers of the 5th British Columbia Coast Brigade stood watch on the lights.[30] Off-duty soldiers befriended the families at William Head, and their support was repaid in kind. As Marjorie Rhode recalled, "thank goodness for their bulging sweaters, which often hid the milk, sugar, and butter they brought for us. It certainly came in handy when the ration book ran out."[31]

In the clear morning of December 25, 1940, those at the William Head Quarantine Station were awakened by the mournful sound of the foghorn at Race Rocks. The lightkeepers and those living at the station had become an extended family, and with the telephone out, the ominous sentinel continued all day. Station staff investigated. It was a cry for help. The lightkeeper had not returned from Rocky Point the night before. Neither his boat nor body were ever seen again, and though parcels and presents for his children were discovered along the shore, Christmas 1940 at the William Head Station Quarantine Station was a time of great sadness.[32]

In 1941, Australian troops who had fought in North Africa were housed briefly at the William Head Quarantine Station while awaiting passage home. Beth Ellwood had become the president of the Metchosin Hostess Club and was able to convince a local wealthy American, Mr. Hunter-Miller, who was at one time secretary to President Woodrow Wilson and had a summer home on Parry Bay, to pay for a bus to bring the soldiers from William Head to the Metchosin Hall for a community dinner and dance. The Aussies, in their best uniformed swagger, thought the whole evening was a "roight good time," and the young women of Metchosin thought all those from the quarantine station were gifts from heaven.

Frustrated Joan Watkins had joined the RCAF (Women's Division) hoping to be posted overseas nearer to her husband. She was sent to Gander, Newfoundland, as a wireless instructor under the Commonwealth Air Training Plan, though within a year she was sent as a signals officer to the RAF Bomber Command base in Linton-on-Ouse, Yorkshire. On leaves, Joan and George met in London, often meeting with Noni and her husband. After the war, the Watkins returned to farm in Metchosin, not far from William Head.

Noni and Tony were separated for only three months during the war, but though he had helped win the Battle of Britain, he could not save the marriage. Noni, childless, returned to Vancouver Island, and as the Fates would have it, married Edward House, a stoker on the *Salucan IV* at the quarantine station. Noni's second marriage lasted ten years. She ended up living with a man who worked at the old ammunitions dump at Rocky Point. Once full of vivacity and promise, in her last few years Noni Bolton was plagued by loss, demons, and men who could not live up to her ventures. Several people at the station who knew her during this dark time reported that she spiralled into despair. Mike Lee said Noni ultimately "drank herself to death."[33]

During the war, many of the wives at the quarantine station, at the urgings of their children, formed a relief organization. They met every fortnight, and received wool, fabrics, and clothing that had been collected by the children from the surrounding communities. They knitted scarves, repaired old clothing, and bundled the whole lot off to the Red Cross to eventually find its way to "their" boys and brothers fighting in Europe.

By the end of the war, enrolment at the quarantine station school had plummeted. Its defining crowd had gone, leaving only three students, Kathleen Rhode, Margaret Taylor, and David Sparks. Margaret's mother, Mrs. Taylor, became the school's last teacher. When high school required these last three to go to Victoria, the school was closed. In 1946, Frank Rhode returned from the war with his war bride and young son. The original schoolhouse became their home.

Diana, Dr. Jenkins's daughter, also married into the armed forces. When Lieutenant Maurice "Migs" Turner of HMCS *Ontario* began courting her after the war, she told him the stories of her friends, of the school, of the beaches, and of the station that played such an important part in her young life. "Migs" listened to Diana and remembered her tales. When he proposed, he took his beloved down to Taylor Beach, sat her upon a log, and, like a knight errant in the wilderness, spoke his piece by the sea she loved. When they married in 1948, half the population of Metchosin and everyone at the station turned out for the wedding. They lived in Victoria, and gracious as ever, live there still today. Diana's father, the good Dr. Jenkins, lived to be over one hundred. His beloved wife, Eve, lived to ninety-nine.[34]

• • •

FROM THE 1920S TO the 1950s, the William Head Quarantine Station was an edifice of stability in an unstable world for western Canada. The children who grew up there during this time countered the station's own class system that initially separated those who worked together. Conditioned by rank and status, the formal organization of life at the station was very clear. "The doctors didn't associate with anybody; then came the captains, customs officers, engineers, and worker bees."[35] The children's idea of institutional life was grounded only in the vitality and brashness of youth, and it softened the station's cool demeanour and broadened its place in the world.

Taken together, the gang became known as the quarantine station's family. They alone crossed the Rubicon. They were an effervescent antidote to the lessons of life that are only learned in blood and tears, and, in their youth, they acted as a vital counter-step to that slide into deference and hopelessness that so often accompanied the ubiquitous presence of disease.

CHAPTER 10 // APOGEE

To strive, to seek, to find, and not to yield.

—Alfred Lord Tennyson, "Ulysses"

On June 13, 1922, a very rich, somewhat overindulged daughter of a prominent New York millionaire began a trip across the Pacific on the maiden voyage of the new *Empress of Canada*. The newly married young woman was en route from Yokohama to Victoria on the latest, most luxurious addition to the fabled *Empress* fleet. With Mother, Papa, and a shiny new husband, Reginald, in tow, she looked forward to staying at the already famous Empress Hotel, seeing the English gardens in Beacon Hill Park, and trying on the latest fashions in the shops along Government Street. A few days before reaching Victoria, the coquettish young bride felt poorly. Had her vaccination not taken? She was pale, developed a fever, and perspired with "the English sweat." As the liner stood off the quarantine station at William Head, she was examined by health officers and diagnosed with a mild case of smallpox. The spanking new *Empress of Canada* was ordered into quarantine, and along with sixty-nine other first-class passengers, she was detained.

Vaccinated and symptom-free, her doting parents and her husband requested to be detained at the station with their darling girl for the full two weeks of her isolation. Separated and believed to be medically protected, her parents and husband were granted many indulgences, and the pampered, cigarette-smoking ingénue sputtered with indignation as she watched her parents and Reginald disappear each morning into the fabled tourist city.

Once in Victoria, it did not take long for the trio to discover that the city not only had an aristocracy, it also had a reputation for fine British goods. After high tea at the Empress each morning, shopping became the norm; the trio went off and bought thousands of dollars' worth of Scottish woollens, Staffordshire china, fine scarves, and expensive prints of bucolic English villages for their swank New York friends and sweets for the young bride who languished alone in isolation.

Her dashing dark-haired husband was a parvenu, a Jay Gatsby character with charm and good looks, who had graduated from the casinos of Monaco. Now, with an assured annual allowance, he was more interested in acquiring silk dinner jackets than in other, more uncertain sybaritic pleasures. Perhaps it was guilt that had him seek out in one small boutique a cloche hat, silk stockings, and a bright red lipstick for his pretty new wife. The *Vancouver Province* estimated "the entire episode [detaining the *Empress of Canada*] ended up injecting about $10,000 [about $100,000], into the Victoria economy."[1] For Victoria and William Head, the Roaring Twenties had begun.

By the mid-1920s, improvements in accommodations and treatment for those detained at the William Head Quarantine Station had changed immeasurably. It was a world away from the one that treated Bertha Whitney in 1872. For the residents of Victoria, the station had once again become a source of pride and Ottawa revelled in its reputation as an integral part of the nation's effective quarantine grid.

In 1919, Dr. Frederick Montizambert, Director-General of Public Health for Canada and one-time superintendent of the quarantine station at Grosse Île, Quebec, wrote:

> *During the past year, at the various stations of the Atlantic and Pacific coasts, 1450 vessels from foreign ports were inspected and 277,910 persons carefully examined. Admissions to hospitals for epidemic diseases were 576. Deaths numbered 55. In every instance, disease was stamped out. Diseases in quarantine did not spread.*[2]

In 1925, G.E. Altree Coley, a reporter for the *Daily Province*, visited the station, anxious to report on its upgrades and innovations. Like Roy

Brown's dispatches in 1900, Coley's copy painted an impressive picture. He described the conditions and procedures at William Head as though they were the bellwether of the Empire's role in the colonies and confirmed that Victoria was still very British in its strict adherence to racial and class distinctions. He began:

> Amid all the busy schemes for securing enduring peace between nations, few people give a thought to the grim menace that forever lurks in the crowded centres of the less-civilized peoples—the menace of epidemic diseases.[3]

Coley was especially impressed with disinfection and fumigation procedures, saying "On the wharf, in place of freight sheds, a long building houses all the appliances for combating infection. Steel rails along the wharf enable the trucks to be pushed by hand to the fumigating plant, where two retorts, each nine feet in diameter, are ready to receive the trucks."[4] He noted the new nine-foot steam-sterilizing chambers were equal in size to the retorts at the quarantine facility at Grosse Île, and its bed count, at least for first- and second-class patients, was actually higher. William Head had arrived. Coley continued:

> Nearby a system of bathrooms takes care of the disinfection of the persons removed from the ship. The bathrooms are now in three separate sections. In the first the individual removes his clothes; in the middle compartment he receives a shower bath, and then passes on to the third where fresh clothing, newly sterilized, awaits him. For women, a dressing room is provided where they may dry their hair and rest after the adventure.[5]

For Altree Coley, the quarantine adventure was constructed from his having seen the facilities available only to the privileged, which he described:

> First-class passengers are given a commodious building having a large central room on each floor, used respectively as a dining room and lounge, from which long corridors extending on either side give access to rooms fitted up much like ship's staterooms. Such equipment

as silver and linen are supplied from the ships, and as stewards accompany the passengers to their detentions, life proceeds very much as on the ship, with the exception that full liberty is allowed only within the confines of the station. Every effort is made by the officials to make the enforced stay as easy as possible, and their gardens and tennis courts become virtually public property.

On every side are to be seen lovely land and sea views. The well-known "Angel's Gateway" in the Olympics reveals dazzling snow-clad peaks, and beyond Victoria, on a clear day, rises the massive dome of Mt. Baker.[6]

Coley waxed poetic over the quarantine station's advances and largely ignored those forced to travel "below the grand saloon." Of his detained and well-off British compatriots, he concluded, "it is not to be wondered at that many involuntary guests have thoroughly enjoyed their sojourn at William Head."[7]

Coley admitted only in passing that Asian detainees, the "steerage inmates," lived in low clapboard dormitory buildings with shelters and "cauldrons for cooking the inevitable rice" until 1923.[8] He discovered, too, that Asian crews of many detained ships all preferred to sleep in the same room "where they have been killing time at gambling."[9] For this reporter, these Asiatic crewmembers at the William Head Quarantine Station "were infinitely better off than their fellow victims in the Orient from whence their diseases were derived."[10] He was right; the William Head Quarantine Station *had* changed, yet the trappings of British superiority remained ubiquitous as ever.

• • •

THROUGHOUT THE EARLY 1920S, the number of ship inspections carried out by medical officers at the William Head Quarantine Station steadily increased. In 1927, ship inspections totalled nearly nine hundred, and the quarantine boats, *Madge* and *Evelyn*, were seldom idle. During these years, both tenders had suffered major damage putting medical officers on board inbound ships in heavy weather. Several of the *Madge*'s hull plates had been smashed from being thrown against ocean freighters during 1923, and the *Evelyn's* deckhouse had almost been ripped off by the winter gales of 1925. It leaked profusely, and on several occasions the *Evelyn* had to be towed to the Esquimalt Dockyard for emergency repairs just to stay afloat. Chief medical officer Chester Brown reported that "both its engine and hull are approaching the limit of safety."[11] Both quarantine boats would soon be replaced.

The numbers of ships inspected at the William Head Quarantine Station increased almost threefold between 1923 and 1927: 285 ships were inspected in 1923; 427 in 1924; 716 in 1925; and 819 in 1926.[12] World trade was on the rise, and ships were inspected twenty-four hours a day. In 1927, 887 ships were inspected and 83,039 passengers cleared.[13] The Chinese Exclusion Act of 1923 did halt Chinese immigration, but the ships kept coming.

By 1927, William Head had become a respected member of an international network of quarantine stations. Dispatches relayed outbreaks of infectious diseases around the world and that expedited control. Dr. Brown reported,

> *Black Plague had been reported from the Straits Settlements at Colombo, Surabaya, Singapore, and Bangkok. There were outbreaks reported from Constantinople, Port Said, and Alexandria, and from Cape Verde in the Canary Islands. Oran and Algiers also reported black plague, while Guayaquil, Callao, Rosario, and Rio de Janeiro in South America, had detected cases of plague upon inspection. Cholera was reported at Singapore, Manila, Hong Kong and Shanghai, but not in epidemic numbers, while typhus was found at Oran, Algiers, and Cairo. It was not surprising that smallpox was reported at almost all ports from which we get traffic.[14]*

During the late 1920s, enhanced radio-telephone equipment further improved the transmission of information among the international quarantine network, and this paid off handsomely for William Head. Of the nearly nine hundred ships inspected in 1927, only two were quarantined for smallpox. One was a passenger ship belonging to the Admiral Orient Line, and the other was a freighter from Europe. On the liner, the ship's surgeon obtained radio information enabling him to vaccinate at-risk passengers such that only one was hospitalized. On the freighter, a crewman had refused vaccination and he, along with another sick crewmember, were immediately detained.

Besides the examination of passengers and crew for suspected contagious diseases, health officers at William Head were required to check all vaccination certificates. To ease the workload, in 1926, William Head adopted "duplicate pratique." It was essentially a clean bill of health certificate obtained for a ship at its port of origin and it enabled health officers to clear a vessel wholesale without time-consuming examination of individual passengers. Upon entering Canadian waters, inspectors examined only the duplicate pratique certificate and, if all was in order, the ship was on its way. By 1935, duplicate pratique became reciprocal between Canada and the United States. In 1937, quarantine officers granted seventy-nine such certificates at William Head and fifty-one on the St. Lawrence. The American quarantine station at Port Townsend, Washington, granted fifty-five such certificates to vessels ultimately destined for Canadian ports.[15] For a time, duplicate pratique certificates were also issued from the islands of St. Pierre and Miquelon and from certain harbours in Panama.

As wireless communication improved during this time, radio pratique further improved the efficiency of the quarantine service. However, the privilege of entering Canada by radio clearance alone was subject to strict regulations. It was not granted to ships from infected ports, was refused to ships with any disease on board, and was refused if a vessel carried cargo that was considered a favourable breeding ground for rats. At the William Head Quarantine Station, radio pratique was granted only to those vessels from Europe via North America, Australasia, and certain Central and South American ports of departure. The risk-filled practice of night-boarding a ship on the Juan de Fuca Strait could be curtailed and replaced by radio clearance. Only in port did a medical officer require to verify radio pratique with written documentation. By 1935, 79 percent of all the entrance procedures were done by radio pratique, followed by shipping traffic in eastern Canada. At William Head, due to infectious diseases being rife in Asian ports, radio pratique was less common.

In 1928, the William Head Quarantine Station cleared the highest number of ocean ships ever inspected since it began its operation; 1,068 ocean vessels cleared quarantine, which was a 20 percent increase over the previous year. That increase was due largely to the increase in numbers of vessels of British and Japanese registry. Ships from Britain accounted for 41 percent of all vessels cleared, and while passenger traffic was down 47 percent, ships' crews increased in number some 15 percent.[16] Economic conditions in Europe changed in the late '20s, and more freighters were required to carry Canadian wheat to Britain and parts of Europe, which suffered unprecedented unemployment. The British coal miners' strikes of 1926 had accomplished nothing except the disintegration of the unions and mass unemployment, making Canadian wheat the one staple affordable for the unemployed. The ensuing demand for cheaper goods increased so much that worn-out British tramp steamers, poorly kept and poorly run, were pressed into service, and they roamed the seas looking for any cargo that might generate some sort of profit. On them, previously uncommon infectious diseases blossomed, especially in the eastern Pacific.

The scare of a new contagion arrived in British Columbia in March 1928 when quarantine officers at the William Head Quarantine Station diagnosed cerebrospinal meningitis among several passengers on three ships of the American-Oriental Mail Line. These ships included those that had repatriated the CLC to China ten years before. Dr. Brown knew that epidemic cerebrospinal meningitis had become prevalent among Filipino steerage passengers and crew travelling from Manila throughout the eastern Pacific that year, so when American-Oriental Mail Line vessels arrived at William Head, the station was already alert to the danger.

Dispatches revealed that Manila had been free from meningitis when the ships left that port, but Dr. Brown learned that the disease was reported in Kobe, Yokohama, Hong Kong, and Shanghai. When the three ships arrived at William Head, the disease had already erupted. Dr. Brown wrote, "It was explosive in character, with a number of Filipino steerage passengers becoming ill during the last day before arrival."[17] Brown discovered that the source of the disease was Asian stewards who carried the infection when they joined the ships in Shanghai. The ships were quarantined.

Meningitis was then a disease of Africa's drier regions and epidemic there in the 1900s. It was rampant in overcrowded villages and market towns of Nigeria and Ghana. It had two forms: viral meningitis, which was less often fatal and was usually cured by ingesting fluids and bedrest; and its counterpart, bacterial meningitis, which was almost always fatal without treatment.

Bacterial meningitis began, like most contagious diseases, with simple flu-like symptoms, but a severe headache was almost always followed by stiffness in the neck. A high fever resulted in intolerance to light, leg pain, involuntary flexing, and periods of lost consciousness. Often, loss of hearing, restricted eye movements, and facial stiffness followed, and in adults, a purple rash was common on the hands. Death occurred from the hemorrhaging of the adrenal glands or from blood pressure that simply fell to zero.

Dr. Brown would have known that bacterial meningitis was an inflammation of the meninges, where meningococcal bacteria from the nasal cavity migrated upward to the protective membranes that enclosed the brain and spinal cord. As bacteria multiplied in the neural tissue, he would have noted seizures and perhaps brain swelling. He might have performed a lumbar puncture with a sick patient lying on his side in order to obtain a sample of cerebrospinal fluid, which then could be examined microscopically for the gram-negative, often twinned bacillus. At the very least, he would have begun a blood culture and done a blood count, but he would not have had access to the C-reactive protein test that is available today. By 1906, a relatively successful anti-serum had been developed but it was unlikely that William Head would have had it on hand. If Dr. Brown's patients miraculously survived without immunization, they faced long-term chronic conditions such as epilepsy, deafness, hydrocephalus, and cognitive impairment. It would take the powerful antibiotics of the 1940s and 1950s to stall the march of this frightening contagious disease.

Other healthy Filipino passengers on the stricken ships were examined carefully and found to be disease free, but Dr. Brown remained cautious. He allowed the ships to dock in Victoria and discharge freight only on the condition that these passengers and their stewards were confined to their quarters. The conditions were met, and the ships were allowed to continue on to Seattle. Those stricken at William Head recovered.

Canadian Pacific Steamships also carried Filipino passengers, so special attention was directed toward the *Empress of Russia* when it arrived in March 1928. Careful clinical and bacteriological examination of those in steerage showed no evidence of cerebrospinal meningitis, but something equally dangerous was about.

Influenzal meningitis had struck several steerage passengers, so Dr. Brown had the whole steerage component quarantined. In total, 318 passengers were detained. By the end of March, eighteen more were hospitalized and two died. During this time, the laboratory at William Head worked overtime. Nasopharyngeal cultures for meningitis were taken from all those quarantined from the *Empress of Russia*. Hospitalized patients were thoroughly examined, and a search for the gram-negative bacillus begun. The spinal fluids turned out to be sterile and free of bacteria,[18] so the outbreak on board the ship, though indeed influenza-like, was viral pneumonia, and despite two more deaths, it had been nipped in the bud.

In late 1928, the chief engineer of a British freighter, seventeen days out from Yokohama, became ill, yet he and his ship passed through examination at William Head. Three days later in Vancouver, he was diagnosed with smallpox, and immediately the ship and its crew were quarantined.[19] Fortunately, they survived.

• • •

Rats!
They fought the dogs, and killed the cats,
and bit the babies in their cradles.
And ate the cheese out of the vats,
and licked the soup from the cook's own ladles.

—Robert Browning, "The Pied Piper of Hamelin"[20]

The William Head Quarantine Station did not need a piper; they had fumigation, and shipping companies were forced to pay handsomely for the service. Rats were everywhere: in ships' holds, in cargo, in steerage, in the galleys, and, at night, even in the first- and second-class saloons. Several first-class passengers on the *Monteagle* or *Empress of Japan* would see them scurrying along the promenade decks when taking their early morning air, as if they had similar entitlements.

With the rats came deadly pathogens. Records revealed that in 1927, the "de-ratization" of 848 ships resulted in the deaths of over four thousand rats. In his annual report, Chester Brown wrote, "684 rats were found on 61 vessels, or 35 percent of all vessels, and each vessel that required quarantine clearance had an average of 11 rats on board."[21] To ease the monthly bottleneck of more than one hundred ships requiring the week-long process, the William Head Quarantine Station created fumigation sub-stations in Vancouver, Victoria, Prince Rupert, and Port Alberni.

Medical officers not only classified the major species of rats found on board incoming ships, they also determined the gender, for both pathogenic and reproductive statistics. It was discovered that male rats generally outnumbered females in a ratio of two to one. As a result, female rats were continually pregnant, while the offspring, from increasingly competitive alpha males, grew more adaptive, aggressive, and cunning with each batch.

All quarantine fumigations on the west coast from 1927 onward were done under the direct supervision of a physician, a medical officer who was appointed by the National Department of Health. By the late 1930s, the Zyklon B cyanide process had become the preferred method of fumigation at the William Head and Vancouver facilities. Because the use of this procedure required highly trained technical personnel, the old sulphur-burning process was used exclusively at the smaller fumigation stations in Victoria, Port Alberni, and Prince Rupert both for safety considerations and as a means of saving money.[22]

However, while William Head Station could order the fumigation process, shipping companies were also required to carry out their own mandatory shipboard disinfections. But of 168 ships fumigated in British Columbia inspection stations in 1929, 93 were charged with failing regular cleaning. When fines began in earnest in 1930, only eleven ships from dis-ease-infected ports were charged and ordered fumigated. By 1931, only five ships had been caught delinquent. As news of British Columbia's hard-line fumigation policy spread, ship owners complied. As well, the names of the offending ships were circulated to quarantine stations around the Pacific, and they were tagged until their agents and owners cleaned up their act.

Before 1931, passenger liners with Asian crews required fumigation after each voyage if they used the old slow-burning sulphur-dioxide process. To offset the delay and expense, quarantine regulations were changed such that ships using the Zyklon B process required only a biannual cleaning. This new regimen was readily adopted, and fumigation-exemption certificates increased in British Columbia ports from 26 to 44 percent after 1931.[23]

There was one other interesting side effect of the Zyklon B process, which affected ships' crews more than any other group that travelled on the freighters and ocean liners of the period. Ships' officers were gener-ally pleased with the outcome of the more powerful cyanide procedure, and reported that its gaseous agent easily killed the abundance of cock-roaches, lice, bed bugs, and other insects found on board. However, crews working the freighters were often negligent in giving their bedding a good airing after it was fumigated by the powerful hydrocyanic gas. On a pas-senger liner, especially in first- or second-class cabins, sheets were regularly changed, and finding a dead cockroach among them was uncommon. On a freighter, old bedding was seldom changed, and the cyanide remained active for several weeks.

A lot of interest was shown in Vancouver and Victoria when Dr. Grubbs of the United States Public Health Service exhibited an improved way of rat-proofing ships that went far beyond the old metal circular rat-guards slung around a ship's mooring lines while in port. However, because the United States still carried out half of all the fumigations done on ship traf-fic during this time, officials in Ottawa refused to make the new devices compulsory. Regardless, the William Head Quarantine Station continued to fumigate ships regularly as part of its quarantine mandate. The statistics speak for themselves:

THE NUMBER OF FUMIGATIONS CARRIED OUT IN COUNTRIES AROUND THE WORLD IN 1927:[24]

United States 351
Canada 102
Japan 73
Great Britain 54
Australia 39
France 30
Germany 27
Holland 12
Cuba 12
Italy 8
Shanghai 6
Hong Kong 2
Brazil 2

The good news for Western Canada that year was that none of the fleas hosted by the fumigated rats were found to be carrying the deadly *Yersinia pestis* bacillus, the causative agent of plague. The bad news was that it cost the William Head Quarantine Station dearly.

On January 9, 1928, Dr. Cox, the assistant medical officer at William Head and Chester Brown's right-hand man, died of injuries sustained in a fall into the hold of the SS *Ethelwulf* as it was being fumigated in Vancouver. Dr. Cox had become Brown's protégé and, for a time, his death sent the station into a tailspin. It took three months to find a suitable replacement, Dr. Cartwright. Then suddenly, at the end of that summer, Dr. H. MacLaren, who had just completed further training in infectious disease control, died of a massive heart attack. Six months would pass before Dr. Brown accepted Dr. Tremayne's experience as being up to the standard of his predecessor's.

During 1928, there were a total of twenty-one quarantine detentions at the William Head Quarantine Station. A virulent form of measles and scarlet fever had been detected among many children whose Caucasian parents had just returned from business postings in Asia in July. Though the adults were not detained at William Head, their children were isolated in several

Victoria hospitals. There were no deaths at the station that year, but one of the measles victims, a young boy, died in an isolation ward in Victoria. He had been diagnosed with scarlet fever and initially quarantined by William Head medical officers, but was later removed to Victoria for an operation. He died from general septicemia following a mastoid infection. The laboratory technicians, station bacteriologist, and medical officers at William Head saw little rest during the peak years, and eternal vigilance would continue to be the rule of the day.

In April 1931, four crewmembers of the freighter *Pretesilaus* inbound to William Head from Shanghai were found sick with yet another flu-like disease. One patient, a Chinese stoker, died soon after being admitted to the station's hospital, and a post-mortem determined that he had died of meningitis. The three others were quarantined, hospitalized, given copious amounts of fluids, and watched. The *Pretesilaus* was duly cleared for Vancouver where it unloaded cargo. Outbound a week later, the three who had recovered rejoined their ship. Vancouver had been saved from an outbreak of viral meningitis, a disease especially virulent among schoolchildren. The quarantine station at William Head was doing its job.

During the early 1930s, keeping ships' crews' vaccinations up to date proved daunting. In May 1931, the *Empress of Asia* arrived at William Head thirteen days after quarantine officials in Kobe, Japan, had detected a case of smallpox on board. Medical officers at William Head found many vaccination certificates among its crewmembers out of date, so a mass re-inoculation was ordered. Canadian Pacific Steamships received a warning from the quarantine service that regulations were being strictly enforced and that heavy fines and imprisonment for both crewmembers and company officials could be imposed. Canadian Pacific Steamships immediately tightened its vaccination-certification policy, and William Head, among shipping agents around the world, gained even more clout.

Chester Brown praised the Japanese quarantine service a year later when they, too, re-vaccinated all on board two ships, the MV *Cressinton Court* and the MV *Bonnington Court*, when each landed a case of smallpox at Yokohama. Japan had adopted the Canadian way. Immediate medical intervention drastically reduced the health risks posed in all international ports. In 1932, Dr. Brown wrote, "Only 44 percent of vessels have brought bills of health showing quarantinable disease as compared to 63 percent last year."[25] The policy of treatment first, followed by warning and investigation later, proved to be most successful.

• • •

IT WAS LARGELY IMMIGRATION to the United States prior to the First World War that had created the golden age of the huge passenger ocean liners. True, the sinking of the *Titanic* and *Lusitania* had shaken the stratified Edwardian society to its foundations, but the great liners, converted into hospital ships and troopships for the duration of the First World War, were back. With oil-fired boilers succeeding coal stokers in the engine rooms, and paint and potted palms replacing soldiers' cots, the big players in the ocean game were again back in business. Cunard's *Mauretania* and *Aquitania*; White Star's *Olympic*; France's *France*; and even Canada's *Empress* fleet had all survived the Great War. Now, the old ocean behemoths, along with some new ones were decked out and gleaming in fresh spit-and-polish, waiting for the money of the Roaring Twenties to roll in. It didn't happen.

In 1921, America changed its immigration rules. The Emergency Quota Act suddenly limited the ingress of people into the United States to 3 percent of a country's national population.[26] In Canada, the Chinese Exclusion Act of 1923 similarly wiped out passenger traffic across the Pacific. Then, America passed one more piece of legislation with as much significance, the Volstead Act.

Prohibition, the "The Noble Experiment," became law in the United States in 1920. For thirteen years, the consumption of alcohol was officially banned in all American territories, and that extended twelve miles out to sea from its continental shores. Worse, all foreign liners were required to padlock their liquor cabinets long before Narragansett Sound or San Francisco hove into view.

For the rich sons of the decidedly affluent smart set, serious drinking was not just a social pastime, it was a duty and an emblem of one's class, and the moniker of privilege. As a result, "Americans avoided their own 'dry ships' and their home ports as if they were, indeed, ships with the plague."[27]

In Canada, prohibition became law in 1917, but it was a provincial issue. Though tough on smuggling, the British Columbia government did not even attempt to prevent anyone from an afternoon's tipple, so stately, well-mannered Victoria doubly reaped the benefits of its post–First World War campaign to ensnare tourists. Not only was the city beautiful, it was also, after 1921, completely "open." For well-heeled Americans, returning directly home to the United States from a voyage across the Pacific was simply out of the question. Such diversions into Victoria would help prop up the doomed fleet of passenger liners until the outbreak of the Second World War. It also helped the local economy.

The largest ship to ever clear quarantine at the William Head Quarantine Station was supposed to be a naval secret until two years after its visit. Just how much of a secret it was remains a moot point. On December 6, 1944, the *Daily Times* released the story. Two years before, on February 25, 1942, the *Queen Elizabeth,* with its massive 83,673-ton bulk, 1,031-foot length, eight decks, and two towering funnels, gently slid into the Esquimalt dry dock. Yarrows Shipyard had been given a job to do, and anyone looking west past Brotchie Ledge toward HMC Dockyard from Victoria would have readily known just what was going on.

The *Queen Elizabeth* was still incomplete in the John Brown and Co. Shipyard in Clydebank, Scotland, in February 1940. The Nazi blitz on London was just hours away, so the admiralty ordered the ship away to sea. The *QE* sped to Singapore and was converted into a troop ship. When the Japanese bombed Pearl Harbor in December 1941, and with Rangoon on the threshold of a Japanese invasion, the whole Pacific Ocean readied itself for a widened global conflict. Undaunted, the *Queen Elizabeth* raced to San Francisco and then just as quickly carried eight thousand American troops to Sydney, Australia. By then, it sadly needed a good cleaning and a refit, and Victoria and the William Head Quarantine Station were the only options. The *Daily Times* reported:

Thousands of bunks were built in any place that could accommodate them. The ship's ornate theatre, its swimming pool, lounges, cocktail bars . . . all became sleeping areas for soldiers packed into tiers . . . The glamorous wainscotings, now soiled, brocaded wall coverings and tessellated floors disappeared. Engines and gear were overhauled . . . High school boys were employed to clean the boilers . . . and 400 sailors from Esquimalt base painted the vast hull.[28]

It was the medical officers from the William Head Quarantine Station who fumigated the massive ship in record time. Within twelve days, the ship was once again ready for sea duty. Clean, reliable, and newly disinfected, the *Queen Elizabeth* carried over 800,000 troops for the duration of the war.

The *News Herald*, as critical as any newspaper during the station's early years, proclaimed just before the Second World War that the William Head Quarantine Station had become "the most commodious station on the west coast."[29] In fifteen years, the station had associated itself with fourteen major steamship companies that operated freighters and passenger liners across the North Pacific and gained worldwide recognition in infectious disease control. The *Daily Times* had proudly proclaimed it "the most up-to-date and best equipped quarantine station in North America."[30] Pilots and sea captains around the world stated that there "was greater efficiency at William Head than at any other quarantine station on the continent."[31] Well past criticism and in its apogee, the William Head Quarantine Station soared in unbounded public acclaim. The accolades had been slow coming, but for those few who knew the station's history, they could appreciate that it was a victory hard won through perseverance, caring, anguish, and blood.

CHAPTER 11 // DÉNOUEMENT

A small town bears the mark of Cain
or the oldest brother with the dead king's wife,
in a foul relation as viewed by sons.
Lies on the land, squat, producing
Love's queer offspring.

—Eli Mandel, "Estevan, Saskatchewan"[1]

D r. Theodore Bain came with what appeared to be solid creden-
tials and strong personal traits. He left Aberdeenshire, Scotland, at
fourteen to join his father, who had immigrated to Canada years
before. Theodore did well in school in Toronto and faced a bright
future when the First World War erupted. He enlisted, and was sent to the
Western Front where he saw mustard gas, trench warfare, thousands dead,
and enough maimed young bodies to beggar the imagination. Somehow,
he survived, returned to Canada, and graduated from the University of
Toronto Medical School in 1926. Then, for five years, he worked with the
Canadian Immigration Service in Glasgow and Edinburgh. That experience was enough for him to be hired as a health officer at the William Head
Quarantine Station in the 1930s. But as self-reliant and accomplished as he
appeared to be, Dr. Bain would soon prove to be woefully inept in dealing
with infectious disease control.

During the 1930s, the number of ships cleared through the William
Head Quarantine Station began a steady decline. In 1931, vessels requesting
clearance dropped by more than one hundred from the previous year, and

the decrease continued. While the Roaring Twenties saw freighter companies replace many of their old tramp steamers constructed at the turn of the century with larger and faster ships, their cargo and passengers shrank as the Depression took hold.

At the same time, the William Head Quarantine Station suffered a downturn in administrative longevity. Dr. Watt, Dr. Nelson, and Dr. Brown had each served for over ten years, and their long experience had given them the confidence to be innovators. They streamlined procedures and developed a network of strong relationships with other quarantine facilities around the Pacific, and their research into treatment of infectious disease control resulted in the station acquiring an international reputation. It wouldn't last.

By 1934, when Dr. Tremayne arrived, ship traffic had shrivelled. In 1936, he inspected only 859 vessels with a total personnel complement of 74,559. Eleven ships were inspected for vermin; nine were given exemption certificates; and two were fumigated.[2] In 1937, only 803 ships were cleared; 733 were boarded; and 70 received radio pratique. After two years, Dr. Tremayne retired. His replacement, Dr. J.S. Douglas, remained acting chief for only six months, until December 31, 1938. Then, on January 1, 1939, Dr. Bain was promoted from within the ranks, and within sixty days the long-standing public acclaim that the station had earned by years of hard work came crashing down.

Just three months before his appointment in October 1938, Dr. Bain addressed the Vancouver Foreign Trade Bureau. Posed on the brink of another world war and hurting still from the economic collapse of the Depression, nervous entrepreneurs wanted to hear that British Columbia was at least safe from epidemics through the protection afforded by William Head. Plain-speaking and severe, Dr. Bain began with a grim picture:

> *If a case of plague were reported in Vancouver, shipmasters, ship owners and quarantine officials the world over would know, within a week, that Vancouver was a plague port. Vessels would avoid us and the resulting financial loss would be enormous.*[3]

But it was all staged. Suddenly, his voice changed, and he boasted of the station's recently installed fumigation apparatus, and commented that it alone would rid any contaminated goods from the deadly pathogens of plague, yellow fever, typhus, and cholera. What Dr. Bain had failed to mention was that the eradication of contagious disease depended more upon the rigorous application of quarantine regulations than upon new technology.

In January 1939, outbreaks of smallpox diseases occurred throughout the eastern Pacific, and Shanghai suffered a particularly virulent epidemic. Though the disease had been tracked by quarantine colleagues around the Pacific, Dr. Bain seemed to have missed the alert. When two ships from that seaport arrived at the William Head Quarantine Station with smallpox on board less than a week apart, a calamity unfolded far more grave than any of Dr. Bain's oratorical predictions.

On February 12, four days away from the station, the captain of the *Queen Victoria* alerted William Head officials that there had been a death on board from scarlet fever. He asked advice from medical officers regarding burial at sea. One particularly astute health officer requested that the body be retained until it could be examined upon arrival. The infection was not scarlet fever, but "hemorrhagic smallpox, and careful examination of the crew revealed one member with a slight elevation of temperature."[4] Even as the ship was tied at the wharf, five more cases of smallpox were developing below decks.

On February 21, 1939, the *Victoria Daily Times* reported that the *Queen Victoria* had suddenly been allowed to proceed to Port Alberni with all hands just six days after being quarantined at William Head. "It is well known," the paper reviled, "that the incubation period of this germ is 14 days or more. Smallpox was in evidence on the vessel when she tied up at William Head from the Orient. As a matter of fact, one seaman had already died of the disease."[5] The people of the Alberni Valley were outraged and wanted to know why the ship was ever permitted to sail in complete disregard of quarantine regulations. Why, they queried, was it not established that the crew was entirely free of disease *before* being cleared? Precautions were undoubtedly taken, the *Times* admitted, "but they do not seem to have been enough to warrant the release of the ship. Why? Who pulled strings, if any? We want to know these things."[6]

The answers never came, because three days later a second ship from Shanghai arrived at William Head, and its story eclipsed the *Queen Victoria* fiasco completely. The news broke in the *Daily Province* on February 28, 1939, and it made the front page:

SMALLPOX PLAGUE STRIKES DOWN 10 AT WILLIAM HEAD.
The British freighter *Rugeley*, a plague ship, lies deserted at the quarantine station dock at William Head, ten miles off this port. Ten of her
crew of twenty-nine are down with smallpox. One of them, William
Woods, third engineer, a Liverpool man, is reported near death.[7]

As chief medical officer, Dr. Bain might have had trouble explaining the release of the *Queen Victoria*, but now he was in it up to his neck. The press eagerly pursued the *Rugeley* story, and the reported horror suffered by its victims put the fear of God in many.

Outbound from Shanghai, the *Rugeley* had sailed for British Columbia in early February to load lumber destined for Australia. On February 14, five days off Victoria, it reported to the William Head Quarantine Station that one crewmember was seriously ill. When the old steamer arrived at William Head on February 19, the sick sailor already showed the telltale pockmarks, and health officers found scabs under the linoleum in the patient's cabin and in the corridor outside. The crew's vaccination certificates were in disarray, and interviews with crewmembers revealed even more confusion. Three had never been vaccinated, nine had been vaccinated in infancy only once, and two vaccinated once in infancy and again later in adolescence. The *Rugeley* was duly quarantined and the patient admitted to the station's hospital.

By February 20, William Woods, the third engineer, was dying; Captain W.H. Hall, Chief Officer F.S. Cummings, Chief Engineer William Sedgewick, and Second Engineer John Litlico were all gravely ill. Within another day, the cook, John Murray, mess-boy Robert Dyas, Steward George Stevenson, and Able Seamen A. Millington and H. Roberts were all stricken. The *Rugeley* had only been in quarantine for twenty-four hours when Millington, Stevenson, and Sedgewick died. The next day, Dyas, Cummings, and Murray died. Within another two days, four more were dead. This startling rise in the number of deaths left the remaining nineteen crewmembers racked with dread. This time reporters pushed harder for an explanation.

Dr. Bain tried his best to mitigate the growing fear. "There is no need for alarm," he said, "and there is no danger of the disease spreading ashore. There have been no contacts."[8] However, the citizens of Victoria were already skeptical of Dr. Bain because of his silence over the *Queen Victoria* incident. As newspapers reported the daily death count, Victoria citizens remembered past smallpox epidemics that had raged unchecked in their city. So palpable was the growing fear that the provincial health officer, Dr. H.E. Young, was compelled to make a statement. He defended Dr. Bain. "I have every confidence in Dr. Bain. The *Rugeley*'s crew is in capable hands. There is nothing to worry the public about. We have the thing in hand."[9]

The truth was that the William Head Quarantine Station had nothing in hand and everything to worry about. Within a two-week period, a total of sixteen cases of smallpox had developed at the station and the death toll was mounting daily. Dr. Young's personal confidence in Dr. Bain was shaken and Victoria citizens readily saw through the charade. Opinion on the street became cynical, more uneasy, and polarized with each passing day. Either this particular strain of smallpox was the most virulent to ever strike this coast, or Dr. Bain had failed to follow basic quarantine practices on two separate occasions. Few believed in the first possibility, and most believed that Dr. Bain's inaction was tantamount to negligence. He had placed their city, and all of British Columbia, at risk.

Throughout that summer and fall, Victoria citizens scrambled to get vaccinated. People distanced themselves from each other, and only a few ventured anywhere near William Head. The *Rugeley*'s owners wanted to send a replacement crew out from Britain, but continuing deaths made a proper count impossible. By the end of September 1939, Victoria shunned Dr. Bain and his staff completely, while rumours at the station were rife with tales of friction among medical officers. The end came quickly. On the evening of Wednesday, October 2, 1939, Dr. Bain slid quietly away from the William Head Quarantine Station, never to be seen again. In an effort to save lives, not to mention the station's reputation, he had unceremoniously been dumped. Dr. Bain had been quietly transferred to Shaughnessy Hospital in Vancouver.[10]

In 1940, Dr. Bain was transferred to Toronto's Christie Street Hospital. In 1941, he moved to Britain and received training in the special care of disabled war veterans. In 1950, he returned to Shaughnessy Hospital, and remained there for fifteen years. Unfortunately, Theodore Bain's métier was not the treatment of contagious diseases. Whether he was the scapegoat for a wider dysfunction at William Head is irrelevant, but the records showed that ordinary quarantine officers were doing meritorious work. The chief medical officer held the supreme responsibility at William Head, and Dr. Bain had failed the community he had sworn to serve. In Veterans Affairs and rehabilitation medicine, however, he would make a positive contribution.[11]

No one was more prepared for the last chapter of the William Head Quarantine Station's story than Dr. Roy Bertram Jenkins. He replaced Dr. Bain, and would be the last chief medical officer at William Head to witness a particular kind of quarantine institutional life in North America. He would restore the station's esteem partly by serving a full twenty years, and, like the energetic Doctors Watt and Chester Brown before him, was a kind and knowledgeable family physician. Bertram Jenkins, however, entered the quarantine service with an established international reputation as a researcher in epidemiology, and he arrived with widespread experience in the treatment of infectious diseases.

The affable, inquisitive, and gutsy Bertram Jenkins had seen it all. His life prior to his appointment in 1939 is significant in that it revealed the calibre of the man well suited to take the station to its end. He was born on the prairies in Carmen, Manitoba, and was in his last year of medical school when the First World War began, so he went overseas and served as a medic in the 1st Canadian General Hospital Corps in northwest France. There, he witnessed the symptomatic, comatose sleep of typhus, the "trench fever" that quietly killed thousands of young soldiers holed up in squalid trenches. There, too, he saw the muscle spasms of tetanus, deadly infections, and the unflagging march of gangrene that preceded crude field-hospital amputations. As conditions deteriorated at the front, the generals sent Bertram Jenkins and some forty other medics back to Canada to finish their medical training. Upon graduation in 1915, he re-enlisted and went to England. He had become interested in infectious diseases and pursued further training at a research station in Epsom, Surrey, where he became involved in the identification of the various strains of viral meningitis. At Epsom, too, he was a part of the scramble to find a vaccine for typhus, the trench disease whose quiet horror had so shaken him a year before.

Jenkins knew that typhus and typhoid fever are completely unrelated diseases caused by different micro-organisms. Typhus is particularly deadly, and its two agents, *Rickettsia typhi* and *Rickettsia prowazekii*, are small virus-like bacteria that multiply only inside host cells. Like diphtheria, typhus is highly contagious, killing hundreds of thousands in the Irish epidemics of 1846, wiping out one-quarter of Ireland's population.[12] It killed over 3 million soldiers in the First World War.

It was carried by lice and fleas on rats and red squirrels, and bloomed in small spaces such as jails, crofts, ships, prisons, concentration camps, and trenches, where overcrowding and squalor reigned supreme. Medics attempting to treat typhus caught the highly infectious disease themselves, as did the commandants, guards, lawyers, judges, and others who oversaw the infected or incarcerated. "Typhus" is a derivative of the Greek word *tûphos,* meaning vapour, smoke, or stupor, and it referred to the trance-like stupor or delirium, the "comatose sleep," that soon overcame its victims. With no treatment in the Great War, the mortality rate was 50 percent.

The disease was characterized by a rash that appeared on the abdomen during the first week, along with fever, chills, and generalized malaise. The rash then spread to the back and chest, leaving the face, palms, and soles of the feet strangely rash-free. As the blood pressure fell, dehydration and septicemia set in, and kidney failure, seizures, coma, and death ensued. If the patient awoke, however, recovery was rapid.

All that Dr. Jenkins could offer to typhus victims at the front in 1914 was a feeble attempt to improve personal hygiene, which included boiling their lice-infected clothing. It was hardly a viable option in the wet of winter with war waging all around. A vaccine for typhus was not found until the mid-1920s, and DDT and antibiotics were not available until after the Second World War. At Epsom, Jenkins learned that strict quarantine was critical in the management of the disease. Typhus was not common at

William Head, but it was at the Grosse Île Quarantine Station in Quebec, where hundreds of Irish immigrants died.

At Epsom, Dr. Jenkins married, and for a moment, life in the time-worn chalk villages of south Surrey seemed safe. But in 1916, he applied for and was granted an officer's commission on the Western Front. Not only did he survive Passchendaele, he turned a bombed-out gun placement into a field hospital where he saved thirty soldiers, Canadian *and* German. For that he was awarded the Military Cross.

Back in Canada, he began his medical practice as a country doctor, administering to sharecroppers in the far-flung farming settlements of central Alberta. It was in Alix, Alberta, that he first saw the signs of the hungry '30s. Most, unable to afford medical insurance, went without treatment, and with their poverty came smallpox, scarlet fever, typhoid, plague, and polio. Of that experience, Dr. Jenkins said, "I used up all my savings looking after the poor."[13]

In the late 1920s, poliomyelitis (infantile paralysis) flared as the economics of the Depression savaged water and sewage systems across the land. No village, town, or city was safe during the summers, and Dr. Jenkins watched helplessly as hundreds of children quietly succumbed. In 1927, he witnessed an Alberta epidemic that resulted in 53 deaths among the 354 reported cases. All that was known about polio at the time was that it was probably caused by a virus. By 1946, 26,000 had been infected across North America, and in 1951, 58,000 caught the disease.[14] It was said that by the early 1950s, Americans' fear of polio was second only to their fear of the atomic bomb.[15]

Dr. Jenkins had kept careful records of the disease among those he served on the rural farms, and in 1928, he took his observations to Alberta's Department of Health. There, his research and suggested treatment of polio gained him national prominence and would lead him directly to the quarantine station at William Head.

He presented the results of an epidemiological survey in a paper submitted to the *Canadian Journal of Public Health* in 1929. He had amassed detailed information on the numbers and movement of family members; cases among schoolmates, friends, and family visitors; the progression of polio's symptoms; and the onset of paralysis. Last, he noted the origins of water and milk supplies. As the categories filled, his hunches about the disease were confirmed. What Dr. Jenkins discovered a full generation before Salk's vaccine became available was truly startling.

The Alberta winter only briefly stalled the virus. When it broke out again in the spring, especially in the north, the outbreaks occurred in completely new areas. Jenkins believed the virus somehow travelled to widely uninhabited areas. He learned, too, that the incidence of the disease was highest among those between the ages of five to fourteen (51.6 percent), affecting only 5.9 percent of those between the ages of twenty-five and forty-four. Those under five years caught the disease in only 19.7 percent of all cases studied. Not surprisingly, 47 out of 189 families revealed two or more cases of the disease within the same family.[16]

Jenkins came to believe that the non-paralyzing symptoms in young carriers was critical in detecting the appearance of the dreaded paralysis. More, he found that paralysis took an average of five days to occur and its route was clear. The onset was gradual, largely gastrointestinal (44.4 percent of cases),[17] and always painful first in the legs. Dr. Jenkins used all this information to shape a treatment. As with typhus, he believed quarantine was the answer, but his proposed kind of quarantine was something very different.

He knew that it wasn't the cold of Alberta's winters that stopped the virus; it stopped only the non-paralytic carriers. When spring returned, many infected young men headed north for work in the oilfields and scattered settlements of northern Alberta. Many, appearing healthy and strong, were on their own for the first time, and Jenkins knew these vigorous young men would not take kindly to being detained in large quarantine facilities. Without expensive security, he knew most would run. He remembered the family solidarity he had seen years before in Alberta's rural hamlets, and considered the less costly idea of home quarantine. Only in home quarantine, he believed, could anxious and caring parents restrict a young man's restlessness as no institution ever could. Moreover, he felt the youngest children of a family could be monitored more directly with an extra, albeit isolated, non-paralytic older brother who remained at home. Jenkins was counting upon the family as a community *within* a community in which siblings, uncles, extended relatives, churches, and other social institutions all played an active role in controlling polio's spread. He was right.

Following Dr. Jenkins's advice, several local health boards throughout Alberta made changes. Schools were closed during spring seeding, and municipalities around Edmonton prohibited young children from being in the streets without a permit. Those under eighteen were not allowed to change their place of residence. For many years after his study, springtime on the high prairies fell strangely silent, not through the dearth of birds, but through the absence of the loud, playful laughter of the young.

Many in the heyday of their youth survived polio, but a few were left with heart-wrenching paralysis. Some 50 percent of those infected faced prolonged medical care, and many would be doomed to the dreaded iron lung. Dr. Jenkins understood that most parents in the 1930s could ill afford such care, and he was instrumental in establishing a sixty-bed special hospital in Edmonton with several outlying outpatient facilities. It opened to all without restriction for a modest nominal fee. In that sense he predated the work of another compassionate man of good faith, who on the whole did not like doctors, Tommy Douglas.[18]

In the mid-1930s, Dr. Jenkins's studies of communicable diseases in Alberta took him to Ottawa as Dominion of Canada Epidemiologist. There, he traced the origins of an outbreak of bubonic plague on the Alberta grasslands to infected fleas that thrived on the gophers living on Alberta's rolling savannah. He discovered that they were being shot and fed to mink by penniless mink ranchers who couldn't afford any other form of food. The ranchers caught the plague as they collected the dead gophers. Jenkins cleared the gophers' habitat with Zyklon B cyanide bombs, and the plague disappeared.

He also discovered plague-infected rats in the Gordon Head area in Victoria. On the Saanich Peninsula, he found that equine encephalomyelitis had entered the bloodstream of farmers from migrating game birds.

In Ottawa, Dr. Jenkins learned of the troubles at William Head and theorized that Bain's problem with smallpox lay in quarantine standards that had been allowed to lapse. When he applied for the position left vacant by Dr. Bain, the station grabbed him. It was a match made in heaven. Immediately, he put strict hygiene and isolation practices into place, and the fearsome outbreak of smallpox disappeared.

But it was in the treatment of leprosy at William Head that Dr. Jenkins truly made his mark. He empathized with the isolation the lepers felt in being forced to spend their lives in confinement, even on idyllic Bentinck Island. Dr. Jenkins spent much of his time there in the early 1940s with the lepers, examining them, probing them, searching for a better treatment.

Familiar with laboratory procedures and methods of microbial staining, Jenkins noted the similarity between the tuberculosis bacillus and the myco-bacterium that caused leprosy. This prompted him to begin a whole new cycle of investigation. He knew that at some hospitals, trials had begun on the bacillus with rudimentary and limited forms of the new antibiotics. If these measures worked on those with TB, Jenkins believed that leprosy might also respond to similar therapy. Taking his cues from research being done at the leprosy centre in Carville, Louisiana, he began an untried clinical procedure.

A young Chinese student studying in Canada had in the 1940s been sent to Bentinck Island with telltale leprous scars on much of his body. With the young man's consent, Dr. Jenkins began to administer isoniazid, the antibiotic tentatively used in the treatment of tuberculosis. Although there was some initial reaction to the drug, the patient's facial scars cleared completely. Jenkins did not publish his findings, because he realized he might have taken undue risks, but in later years he felt he should have, in spite of possible censure. Though he had actively extended the life of one leper, he regretted not influencing more physicians through publication of his research. At the time, he justified his caution with the belief that the last thing the William Head Quarantine Station needed at this juncture was more controversy.[19]

Roy Bertram Jenkins was a pragmatist. If he could not introduce a new large-scale antibiotic treatment for the lepers on Bentinck Island, he would contribute to their well-being. As international shipping through William Head almost stalled during the Second World War, Jenkins secured extra personnel and an isolation facility for the Bentinck Island Leprosarium.

···

THE ONE PROCEDURE THAT grew during the Second World War was the de-ratization of troopships and warships of the Navy through regular fumigation. Soon after the war, the port of Vancouver regained prominence, and freighters with rats on board showed up in growing numbers, as revealed in the following table:

VESSELS FUMIGATED IN WILLIAM HEAD/VICTORIA/ ESQUIMALT AND VANCOUVER 1945–1951[20]

YEAR	FUMIGATIONS AT SUB-STATIONS	FUMIGATIONS AT VANCOUVER
1945–46	3 at Victoria/Esquimalt	36 at Vancouver
1946–47	0 at Victoria/Esquimalt	82 at Vancouver
1947–48	4 at Victoria/Esquimalt	44 at Vancouver
1950–51	1 at Victoria/Esquimalt	59 at Vancouver

The fumigations decreased at William Head's sub-stations, and they were closed in 1948. The Victoria fumigation sub-station was shut down in 1951.

The last ship to undergo fumigation at the William Head Quarantine Station was the Canadian destroyer/escort HMCS *Athabaskan* in 1948. On board, Dr. Jenkins found more than rats; he found the likelihood of polio. When the warship arrived at William Head in late summer en route to Esquimalt, Jenkins established that the ship had been on diplomatic and military manoeuvres on the east coast and had visited New York City. Knowing that a polio epidemic waged there at the time, he questioned the crew in great detail. It became evident that many on shore leave had visited boroughs of the city where the disease had struck, and there was a high probability that some might have been infected by non-paralytic carriers. Without flinching, Jenkins took what appeared to be very dramatic action for the navy. He quarantined the ship, detained everyone on board, and had the ship fumigated. The admiralty raised their eyebrows at detaining naval officers and crew alike, but Jenkins did not care. Before the sputtering could begin in earnest, he had every mattress on the ship brought ashore and fumigated again. Then he told the navy brass and the press just what he had done. During the summer of 1948, Victoria remained polio-free. As the end neared for William Head, most realized that Ottawa had, indeed, appointed the right man.

The Second World War had irrevocably altered trade and travel patterns across the Pacific. Those who worked at the station and recalled the zenith of its activities years before knew it was over. Percy Gray had been the chief steward at William Head for over thirty years, and he held onto the belief that a flurry of post-war activity was a sign of better things to come. "By April of 1947," he wrote, "394 ships have already been inspected, and world shipping is once again beginning to open up."[21] Roy Bertram Jenkins, though hopeful, was a little more stoical. "Things were a little slow during the war and that increased traffic would actually be welcome."[22]

• • •

BY THE END OF 1948, the William Head Quarantine Station had become too large to sustain. Built to detain more than one thousand individuals with state-of-the-art laboratory, fumigation, and isolation facilities, and four inshore launches standing ready to roar out onto Juan de Fuca Strait at a moment's notice, it was now virtually motionless. In the last nineteen years of its operation, Dr. Jenkins reported that although incoming vessels *were* still inspected for infectious diseases twenty-four hours a day, "we only took two [sick] people off the ships in all that time, so it was a rational, sensible decision to close up that service which cost the taxpayers quite a bit each year. When I recommended the closure, I wasn't very popular because I didn't help them out to spend their money in Ottawa."[23]

By 1952, it had become common knowledge around Victoria that the days of the William Head Quarantine Station were numbered. For those on-site, the signs were everywhere. The hospital and detention quarters had remained empty for years, and Dr. Jenkins had become little more than an expensive customs officer. Indeed, when he retired in 1956, his replacement, Dr. Stanley Blundell, although a physician, was a man with years of overseas experience in the Canada Customs Service. The imminent closure of the station not only brought into question the future use of its extensive facilities, it also raised the issue of the kind of quarantine facility that might be required in the changing post-war world that was taking to the skies.

The first tangible alternate use of the William Head site came from the federal government. On November 20, 1954, Robert Bonner, British Columbia attorney general, received a letter from Federal Health Minister Paul Martin. His proposal for a drug addiction treatment centre at William Head made the front pages.[24]

Clearly delighted by his brainwave, he wrote, "the Station which is now little used because of the rarity of communicable diseases aboard visiting ships, would be moved to another location."[25] He backed his idea with money. "The province could get federal financial assistance also, under the policy whereby Ottawa pays grants to hospitals at the rate of $1,000 a bed."[26] Carefully eyeballing the electorate, Attorney General Bonner was only lukewarm and demanded a conference of ministers. The debate waged in the local papers.

Bonner understood the growing "not in my backyard" concerns of Victoria citizens and felt they had had enough. After years of having an established quarantine edifice in their midst, Bonner believed the local population strongly opposed another so-called rehabilitation institution on their doorstep. In response to Mr. Martin's offer of money for a drug-treatment centre, Bonner presented an image of crazed addicts prowling Victoria's historic streets. He knew, too, that British Columbia already operated a drug-addiction program at Oakala Prison on the mainland. If any duplication was deemed necessary, then Ottawa's proposal, Bonner suggested, should be located near Vancouver, "where almost all of the BC addict population is located."[27] Victoria citizens, remembering old rivalries, cheered. The issue was dead.

In 1954, it was learned that the provincial government had considered that the old quarantine station be used as an emergency "shelter" for British Columbia Doukhobors who were arrested after the violence and nude marches made by the Sons of Freedom sect in the East Kootenays. It came to nothing.

Private developers became interested when it was leaked that the adjacent Bentinck Island Leprosarium would be closed at the same time as the quarantine station. The island was one of the most beautiful on the coast, and some entrepreneurs thought the old leper colony might easily be transformed into a magnificent high-end resort. But a citizens' survey revealed that the fear of recurring leprosy endured, and its location near an institution with a long-standing history of infectious diseases hampered the proposal. The developers turned to look elsewhere.

In 1957, the real fate of the William Head Quarantine Station became public knowledge. The *Daily Times* stated that it would be downsized and moved into the old immigration building in Victoria and the buildings on the site would be turned over to the Crown Assets Disposal Corporation (CADC) for disposal.

This prompted the Victoria–Esquimalt Board of Health to ask Ottawa for a long-term lease of the buildings for use as a district mental hospital. Board officials felt they could be used "as a home for senile persons for whom there are at present no adequate nursing home facilities in this area."[28] The health board was told in no uncertain terms that when the buildings were declared surplus, "you will be given the opportunity to acquire the property. However, the CADC sale would likely go to the highest bidder, as government policy is to sell by tender." The health unit backed away from the proposal, refusing to enter a bidding war with public money.

It was Dr. Jenkins who came up with one of the wisest proposals for the future use of the William Head site. He, along with others in the surrounding communities, began a campaign to turn the site into a "first-class federal or provincial park."[29] Jenkins knew of the rejuvenating power of the natural beauty of its high peninsula with its undulating lawns, stands of trees, beaches, and magnificent views across the strait. He even felt that the old brick buildings should remain within the park, providing palliative care accomodation for the chronically ill. Though the campaign came to naught, Dr. Jenkins, ever the healer, had become suspicious of new certainties. He said, "While we don't need an establishment such as William Head any longer, we always keep our fingers crossed that infectious diseases won't return with a vengeance."[30] Little did he know just how prophetic his words were.

In November 1958, "The planning committee of the [Federal] Justice Department decided, rather than scrap the buildings, to use part of William

Head's facilities to relieve overcrowding at the BC Penitentiary."[31] The penitentiary located in New Westminster already held some two hundred more inmates than it was originally designed for, and such overcrowding, it was touted, would lead to violence. The operative word in the Justice Department's plan was the word "part," but they did not reveal the extent of the buildings at William Head, which were to be co-opted. The British Columbia Penitentiary Service assured a skeptical population that what they had in mind was an absolutely "open" minimum-security prison. The only fence, they promised, would be one constructed to "keep out gawkers."[32]

Planned initially as a pre-release centre, the new facility was to have "no bars, no cells, and no high stone walls."[33] They promised the site would have no on-site administration and few rules for its convicts. Posing no danger, the reduced quarantine service could, they argued, safely continue to use unoccupied buildings. Ottawa became firm. Much of the old William Head Quarantine Station would become a prison.

That was the plan, and for a short time it worked. On January 9, 1959, the first three inmates arrived at William Head, escorted by four guards, two cooks, and a plumber's helper. On January 16, the number of inmates had increased to twenty-five, and by the end of the month, it had risen to fifty-five.[34] It did not take the inmates long to discover that the peninsula was not only naturally beautiful, it was also one of the best fishing spots in North America. On February 1, 1959, it was reported that a five-foot octopus was caught at exactly the same location where CLC members had pulled a similar creature from the ocean some forty years before. Prison officials concluded that such activities were just too much fun for inmates, so strict rules immediately took effect. The old railing to keep out gawkers was to be replaced with a very high fence.

On March 5, 1959, the Department of National Health officially transferred thirty-five acres of land from the William Head Peninsula to the Department of Justice. The remaining seventy-one acres continued to be used as a quarantine facility for a short time, but even that would not last. Dr. Blundell, soft-spoken, alert, and methodical, was determined to carry out Ottawa's larger wishes. On July 9, 1959, The *Daily Times* carried the news:

OLD QUARANTINE STATION MOVING

The Quarantine station which has operated at William Head since 1894 will move into the Canada Customs Building, formerly the post office, ready for service August 2.[35]

Dr. Blundell explained what was already known to many. He claimed that the formation of the World Health Organization (WHO), with its international "eyes" had resulted in decreased quarantine activity worldwide. He reiterated that local ship inspections, which were still a worthy means of defence against the introduction of infectious diseases into British Columbia, would continue. However, Blundell also stated that the station's staff, then already reduced to fourteen, would be cut further. The *Times* continued, "Certain posts were to be eliminated and employees absorbed into other branches of the service. The quarantine service will get rid of its own vessels and use the BC Pilotage Authority craft [stationed at] Dallas Road."[36] Quarantine officers would board inbound ships from an anchorage near Albert Head. The present move, the paper continued, "will be desirable for the penitentiary which can take over all the property."[37]

So Dr. Blundell had become the hatchet man of the old quarantine institution. Officially, he claimed that the shift of activities from William Head to Government Street in Victoria was to keep civilians from living in close proximity to prisoners of the state. Unofficially, immigration and not quarantine had become Ottawa's new mantra. Papers reported, "There will be a slight delay in relocating some of the station's families in the city, and a certain amount of equipment and stores will be left behind at William Head for disposal later."[38] Like the remains of the old Inuit outposts in the High Arctic after resettlement, the leftover structures of the quarantine station would be left to the weather. The wharf, to which the white *Empress* fleet once tied, would rapidly fall into ruin. The iron rails to the fumigation sheds that were once full of passengers' baggage and clothing would rust, and the myriad of pipes in the steam boilers would house new populations of rats. Cobwebs would reign in the isolation hospitals, while the first- and second-class passengers' quarters morphed into prison accommodation. It was over.

Chris Rhode was a boy of nine in 1925 when he arrived at William Head. He worked at the station for thirty-four years and was its last assistant engineer. He served in the quarantine service for the same number of years that his father, Frank, had years before. Chris, fondly nostalgic for the station's more useful time, stated, "Smallpox was a big deal in those days. We all stayed home for three weeks, sometimes six. The gates were locked and all supplies were brought in by steamer. Now, smallpox is a thing of the past."[39]

Mike Lee, who had worked at the quarantine station for over ten years, was offered a position as a guard at the new William Head Penitentiary. He disliked working for the prison service, maintaining that it was too full of administrative bullying and bureaucratic deceit. The real reason that the old quarantine inshore tenders were finally sold, Mike stated, wasn't Blundell's chopping, "it was because a few minimum-security prisoners had taken the alcohol from the compasses in the boats' wheelhouses and got drunk."[40] Mike retired early.

When the William Head Quarantine Station closed in 1959, the word "quarantine" was fast disappearing from the English language. The Ellis Island Quarantine Station had closed in 1954, and Canada's first national quarantine station at Grosse Île, Quebec, had closed in 1937. The Halifax Quarantine Station on Lawlor's Island closed a year later. By the 1960s, America had only fifty-five institutional quarantine stations left, and by the 1970s, the old quarantine system, as it once stood, had been dismantled.

The era that ended in 1970 had been a time of unqualified faith in the miracle of science. Man had just landed on the moon, the code of the double helix had been unravelled, and computer technology pointed to a brave new world. Improvements in medicine, especially in the use of antibiotics, made quarantine stations and infectious diseases relics of the past. The old guardians of the nation state, once bastions of and gateways to the hoped-for disease-free new world, had done yeoman service. Suddenly they were declared obsolete. The Center for Disease Control made the call in 1968, reporting, "it was time to close the book on infectious disease, declare the war against pestilence won, and shift national resources to such chronic problems as cancer and heart disease."[41] They could not have been more wrong.

Dr. Jenkins, however, understood that the battle against infectious diseases would never end. He had witnessed microbial adaptation, and was amazed by the virulence and resilience of the pathogens he sought to tame. "Quarantine may evolve," he stated, "but it is certainly not over."[42] Even his successor, Dr. Blundell, though from a new tradition of the civil service, believed that the need for quarantine detention in some form would remain. "The job has changed," he said, "and in many ways it has become more difficult with air travel."[43] How right the predictions of these two men would turn out to be.

CHAPTER 12 // QUARANTINE REVISITED

They won't let us out!

—Yuri Ivanov to Scott Percival in John Erick Dowdle's film *Quarantine* (2008).

D r. Blundell said that it would come from the skies, and like the wrath of some vengeful god, it did. The return of the microbes began long before the gates of the William Head Quarantine Station were dismantled. Paradoxically, their recurrence was enabled by both war and peace, and expedited by two airplanes, the B-29 Superfortress and the Lockheed C-69 Constellation.

The B-29 came into its own during the final years of the Second World War. This heavy-payload, four-engined bomber pummelled Japan in the fire bombing of Tokyo and dropped the atomic bomb on Nagasaki in August 1945. After the war, the B-29 Superfortress evolved into the Boeing Stratocruiser. Boasting the capability to travel from New York to Hawaii in less than twenty-four hours, Pan American Airways and Northwest Orient Airlines were using the squat, double-decker, long version of the Stratocruiser on their regularly scheduled air service across the Pacific by 1956.

The C-69 entered the latter stages of the war as a military transport airplane but its speed gave it strength as a reconnaissance and airborne-detection aircraft in the Cold War. Lockheed Constellation's "Connie," with its distinctive triple-tail and thin, dolphin-shaped body, soon caught the attention of the public. By 1953, BOAC (British Overseas Airways Corporation), Air France, Lufthansa, and Trans-Canada Airlines were operating fleets of Connies on daily flights across Europe, Africa, and the Atlantic.

During the post-war boom, both these piston-driven aircraft morphed into long-range passenger planes that opened the skies for millions of new peacetime travellers and their not-so-friendly parasites. They would change quarantine history completely.

In the 1950s, shipping magnates and corporate managers of the old ocean liners quibbled over the distinctions between the new "tourist cabin class" and "tourist third class" in an attempt to entice a new generation of youthful travellers to a slower, more socially stratified time. Stuck in the mentality of travel within a rigid class system, ocean passages of this sort were doomed. The rich post-war college-set were no longer interested in squashing a dinner jacket or an evening dress into their new lightweight backpacks. When Alvin "Tex" Johnston did two barrel rolls over Seattle in a Boeing 707 jetliner on August 7, 1955, the operators of the old ocean fleets knew the gig was up. The dinosaurs of the deep had become extinct, and the new pterodactyls had taken wing. The Jet Age, the age of fast and affordable air travel, had begun in earnest, and microbes and people had found a new way to fly.

• • •

THE AIRBORNE DISEASES THAT were initially feared were yellow fever and malaria. Experiments in Africa before the war revealed that mosquitoes stowed among baggage could survive aircraft journeys of over nine thousand miles. As a result, in 1947, all passengers flying over endemic yellow fever zones were required to present current vaccination certificates. Increasing document forgery and spotty dusting with noxious pyrethrum led Dr. G.M. Findlay, consulting physician to the West Africa Command, to argue successfully for the WHO to take charge of aircraft pesticide control and air-passenger vaccination certification.[1] It didn't help.

It took less than thirty years for strange micro-organisms to be fully disseminated around the world. During that time, the gains that antibiotics had made against infectious diseases were already being eroded through an evolutionary phenomenon called drug-resistance. It was noticed first in the treatment of malaria.

Just before the Second World War, an inexpensive new drug, chloroquine, was developed to fight malaria. It was used widely in the post-war years, and by 1948, it was considered the most successful organic compound ever deployed against the disease. It was used in concert with DDT and the mass spraying of mosquito habitats, and the WHO felt confident that by 1955, chloroquine would eradicate malaria worldwide.

Within twenty years, the drug was useless. By the late 1960s, malaria's causative agents, *Plasmodium falciparum* and *Plasmodium vivax,* had become totally resistant to chloroquine in South America, Southeast Asia, and India. By the 1970s, those in Central Africa still taking the drug showed no improvement.[2] In one generation, the curative qualities of chloroquine were no more as pathogens simply followed the ceaseless practice of adaptation. Along with the old agents of smallpox, cholera, tuberculosis, typhus, bacterial meningitis, and polio, which stood lurking in the wings, new contagions arrived from places whose names we hardly knew how to spell. Without visa or passports, swine flu, Lyme disease, E. coli, Creutzfeldt-Jakob disease, West Nile virus, the deadly hantaviruses, Ebola, AIDS, SARS, and untold new influenzas had all landed and demanded a new status that simply could not be dismissed. Hubris and complacency had let them in.

It began in earnest in 1981. A report from the Center for Disease Control and Prevention in New York described "a strange cluster of fatal symptoms among five gay men in Los Angeles they called acquired immunodeficiency syndrome or AIDS. It had already silently infected 250,000 in the United States."[3] The appearance of HIV/AIDS in North America's gay communities of Los Angeles and San Francisco signalled the beginnings of the new worldwide pandemics. It blindsided health professionals and re-created a climate of denunciation and hysteria not seen since the onset of the black plague in the quarantine cities of the old world.

When HIV/AIDS hit, it was a *Heart of Darkness* moment. The West's post-colonial superiority complex was challenged, its moral roots shaken, and its anthropocentric view was cast into oblivion. A new and uncontrollable epidemic was among us, and the fear was palpable.

From the first moment the casualty count of HIV/AIDS began to soar, the world uttered a collective gasp. Even in the light of swine flu and legionnaires' disease, here was a drug-resistant, full-fledged plague right in our midst. In an instant we were taken aback by an overwhelming sense of incredulity, so soon it was since the scientists had defeated polio! With no cure, violence struck out against African-Americans, homosexuals, and even the monkeys. It was as if we had, all over again, debated Darwin and his dastardly idea of evolution. Suddenly we were just animals that caught germs from other animals. Moral astonishment readily turned into moral outrage. What a clever monkey!

In America, those with HIV/AIDS were initially "shunned and evicted from their homes, fired from their jobs, and kept out of schools. Not surprisingly it was the marginalized groups; the blacks, gay men, intravenous drug-users, and immigrants, especially from Haiti, that bore the brunt of the fear and antipathy."[4] It did not end there. HIV-positive individuals were banned from entering the American army and foreign service until 2009, and HIV-positive Haitian refugees were removed to Guantanamo Bay long before it became a detention centre for alleged terrorists. The Reagan administration banned travel by HIV-infected foreign nationals to the Sixth International AIDS Conference in San Francisco in 1990; excluded non-resident would-be participants worldwide sought legal action. Though most of the restrictive and prejudicial measures were largely overturned by US federal courts, the National Department of Health and Human Services in Washington, DC, is still able to deny entry into the United States to any person with an excludable disease such as AIDS.[5]

• • •

IN NOVEMBER 2002, THE public health agency in Canada posted a report on its Global Public Health Intelligence Network (GPHIN), stating that "an unusual number of people were showing up in an emergency room in Guangdong, China, suffering from what looked like atypical pneumonia."[6] On February 9, 2003, a teacher in Fremont, California, passed on to a physician-friend in Maryland an Internet chat-room message that claimed so many were stricken that a hospital in Guangdong had locked its doors. The physician alerted ProMED-mail (Program for Monitoring Emerging Diseases), "a global electronic reporting system for outbreaks of emerging infections and toxins."[7] ProMED staff alerted its worldwide clientele, and the next day the WHO, a major subscriber, issued a bulletin. SARS had arrived.

When SARS appeared in North America in 2003, the WHO finally woke up. SARS was yet another xenographic virus that crossed the animal-human barrier from monkeys to man. In the case of SARS, it was believed the virus moved from cats, raccoons, bats, and possibly badgers to humans. This corona virus was totally unaffected by antibiotics, though it was partially controlled by antipyretics, drugs that reduce body temperature such as acetylsalicylic acid, acetaminophen, and ibuprofen. Yet, such drugs only helped to prevent or alleviate fever.

More significantly, the SARS pandemic would kill 774 people and infect more than eight thousand others in twenty-seven countries.[8] Health officials once again called for the reintroduction of strong quarantine measures. By March 17, 2003, authorities in Hong Kong decided to screen airline passengers for symptoms of SARS, and a month later, thermal imaging began to be used to scan international travellers in Changi airport in Singapore. By April, 2003, twelve hundred persons with SARS had been quarantined in Hong Kong and approximately one thousand more were quarantined in Singapore and Taiwan. In 2003, Toronto suffered forty-two deaths from SARS. Local boards of education considered closing the schools for a period of up to ten days, and several large public gatherings were cancelled.

New quarantine regulations prohibited those with SARS from being in public places, and isolation wards in hospitals tried, unsuccessfully, to restrain many more. In some countries, the hastily adopted regulations also levied fines, imprisonment, and electronic wrist-tagging for those who ignored the stay-at-home quarantine restrictions. Prosecution was also enacted to deter those who were proven to have lied about having caught the disease.

A highly pathogenic avian influenza (bird flu) struck Southeast Asian countries in 2004. In Canada, the *Toronto Star* reported that since the morphed H1N1 strain emerged in April 2009, 8,102 people have been hospitalized, and 390 people have died from the disease. Dr. David Butler-Jones, head of the Public Health Agency of Canada and Canada's first chief public health officer, reported in December that year that vaccination remained the best possible measure against the onset of the disease. Though the disease turned out not to be as virulent as first feared, Jones reasoned that a dangerous third wave of the rapidly evolving virus was then still possible.[9] In Australia, the impact of an influenza pandemic *without* the use of an effective vaccine had been assessed as capable of causing 13,000–44,000 deaths.[10]

During the late spring of 2011, a massive outbreak of E. coli O104 had infected 1,800 people in Europe and left some 500 more with a life-threatening urinary complication called haemolytic-uremic syndrome. The infection raced across the borders of thirteen countries and killed twenty of its victims. E. coli O104 had become resistant to "more than a dozen anti-biotics in eight classes."[11]

But investigators found a strange anomaly in that antibiotics were *not* normally used in the treatment of E. coli infections, and when given, "caused toxins to be released which brought on the illness's worst symptoms."[12] However, if antibiotics were *not* used, and the vast overuse of antibiotics worldwide was a major factor in the development of drug-resistant pathogens, what caused E. coli O104 to become immune to antibiotics in the first place?

The answer, researchers found, lay in the way that pathogens had learned how to leap-frog their drug-resistance genes into new micro-organisms, which were previously susceptible to pharmaceutical intervention. It seemed that viruses and certain bacteria had developed an evolutionary strategy that enabled them to pass on drug-resistant factors to other related micro-organisms that previously yielded to antibiotic therapy. In the 1990s, "a drug-resistant strain of Klebsiella, a bacterium that causes serious hospital-acquired infections began ping-ponging its way through Europe. Initially, Klebsiella infections were limited to patients hospitalized in intensive care units and posed no danger to the general public."[13] After 2001, these same resistance factors suddenly appeared in other pathogens of everyday life, including some strains of E. coli.[14] When a woman, unresponsive to antibiotics, died of a Klebsiella infection in North Staffordshire, England, in 2010, not only had Klebsiella become deadly outside hospitals but the related E. coli O104 bacterium had simultaneously begun its new assault. Drug-resistant pathogens had come of age in a time when old quarantine narratives of ships and the sea were almost forgotten.

The sleek coal-burning ocean liners of *La Belle Époque* that carried hundreds of thousands of immigrants to our shores had by the 1970s, evolved into the cruise ship phenomenon. These meandering matronly gin palaces for the white-haired gambling set had become the new rage. With them on the dining tables, in the drinks, in the salads, and in the desserts came the Norwalk virus. In May 2007, 130 cases were reported on the *Norwegian Star*. Then in November that year, three hundred passengers became ill on the *Queen Elizabeth 2*. In December, on the maiden voyage of Cunard's *Queen Victoria*, 135 passengers were stricken, and in January 2008, a Carnival Cruise Lines sojourn to Cozumel, Mexico suffered an outbreak of 143 cases of the Norwalk virus.[15] Frighteningly, though a member of the gastroenteritis-causing group of noroviruses, Norwalk is not always transmitted in food and, though an attack of the virus is not life-threatening, it often causes severe bouts of nausea, vomiting, diarrhea, chills, and muscle pain—enough to ruin any cruise-ship sojourn completely.

With Reagan's deregulation of the aviation industry in the mid-1980s and the European Union's similar action in 1992, the skies suddenly opened to "no-frills" air carriers such as People Express and Ryanair. A new global market had been laid bare and cheap flights to Bangalore or Lhasa enabled the young and reckless to flock to more remote parts of the world in numbers approaching that of the migration of butterflies to Brazil. Too often their blood, infected from a mosquito bite in Cairo, spread dengue fever far afield as the young adventurers moved easily from Amritsar to Agra.

On November 5, 2011, the *Hindustan Times* reported 337 deaths from dengue fever during past the year in Lahore, the capital city of the Pakistani province of Punjab. Thirty thousand more had been infected. With young passengers eager to explore the most inaccessible and penniless parts of the planet along with untold drug-resistant pathogens, discount airlines stood to morph into the new "coffin ships" of our time.

• • •

ON AUGUST 9, 2007, Health Protection Scotland quarantined a flight from the Dominican Republic at the Glasgow International Airport when norovirus was detected among sick travellers.[16] On September 23, 2007, the Centers for Disease Control and Prevention in Washington, DC, quarantined passengers on a flight from Australia to Hawaii when ten became ill. It was determined later that the infected passengers had only suffered from food poisoning. On November 13, 2007, New Zealand health authorities quarantined 223 people on a flight from Korea by way of Australia when a woman on board exhibited symptoms of the flu. She was later found to be suffering from gastroenteritis and deemed no risk. In March 2008, a plane en route from the Dominican Republic to Canada was directed to make an emergency landing in Florida when several passengers complained of illness. The cause was never identified though the Centers for Disease Control officials declared it not contagious.[17] These bouts, contagious or not, had quarantine officers around the world fast becoming rightly nervous. Old fears had become new again.

Following Dr. Findlay's lead, and in response to the 2009 H1N1 flu epidemic, Health Canada published its own simplified Civil Aviation Contingency Plan for Pandemics and Communicable Disease Events. It designated six airports in Vancouver, Calgary, Toronto, Ottawa, Montreal, and Halifax as quarantine sites, with three (Toronto, Montreal, and Vancouver) charged with meeting all emergency requirements as required by international health regulations. In addition, fifteen additional Canadian airports were listed, "where a person in charge of an aircraft arriving from outside Canada must alert a quarantine officer if they wish to land."[18]

Just as it is the obligation of a ship's captain to report sickness to a quarantine officer upon arrival at an international port, it is the responsibility of an airline pilot to make a similar declaration. The captain's task is still stringent and carefully laid out in Canadian Quarantine Regulations, CRC, c. 1368. Subsection 19 bears repeating:

AIR TRAFFIC

19. **(1)** Where a person in charge of any aircraft arriving in Canada from a place outside Canada wishes to land at any of the airports listed in subsection **(2)**

(a) he shall, prior to arrival, except in cases of emergency or other circumstance in which it is impossible to communicate with the airport, send by radio to the quarantine officer at such airport information concerning

(i) any illness among the persons on board the aircraft, other than air sickness, or resulting from any accident that might have occurred during the flight, with detail of such illness including the existence of fever, skin rash, headache, backache, jaundice, diarrhea, vomiting, chills, or abnormal behaviour, or

(ii) the death of any person on board the aircraft during the flight: and

(b) he may, where no illness described in subsection (a) (i) has become apparent and no death has occurred during the flight, send by radio to the quarantine officer at each airport a message that all on board appear to be healthy.[19]

There are twenty-one airports in Canada licensed to land international traffic and each has a designated quarantine officer available to screen passengers for suspected contagious disease. According to the International Air Transport Association (IATA) statistics, Toronto's Pearson International Airport (YYZ) handled over 30 million passengers in 2009. The same year, Vancouver International Airport (YVR), had over 16 million pass through its gates. Of these, at least one-quarter were international travellers, all highly mobile and, often through the demands of business, very socially interactive.

In America, in 2009, Lufthansa carried 42 million international passengers; Air France carried 32 million; and British Airways and Cathay Pacific combined carried over 47 million international fliers. Each one of them, somewhere, stood patiently in line, breathing another's air, eager to board and get through customs. One single sneeze amongst such numbers could, statistically, spread enough contagion that would readily overwhelm any quarantine facility. The WHO understood the gravity of the situation when it stated, finally, "infectious diseases are now spreading geographically much faster than at any time in history."[20]

Dr. Jenkins and Dr. Blundell had been right; the germs were back with a vengeance. The old quarantine stations of the past just barely evolved in our cost-effective culture into small offices within major international airports housing less than a half-dozen public health officials.

In 2006, at O'Hare International Airport, one of America's largest air terminals, the quarantine unit was one such office located near customs. With one administrative officer, one quarantine medical officer, four public health officers, and two assistants, they faced the daunting task of protecting the public from infectious diseases at an airport "that saw 5,055,987 international arrivals that year."[21] Even in its best times, the William Head Quarantine Station with four times the staff could never handle what analogously amounted to 620 international arrivals per week.

In Canada, the situation is similar, though its efficacy is a little harder to assess. Currently, there are nearly two dozen quarantine officers posted in designated airports across Canada along with administrative personnel. Most officers are registered nurses with special training in infectious diseases and federal quarantine legislations. There is also one quarantine director (a physician) based in Ottawa and two quarantine officers (also physicians) based in Toronto and Ottawa. There are six "quarantine stations" across Canada, located at international airports in Vancouver, Calgary, Toronto, Montreal, Ottawa, and Halifax. Each of these stations has a station manager, who, besides keeping records, is a registered nurse.

Passengers who might be healthy but are suspected of being carriers of contagion are simply "held" on arrival by airport officials. The word "quarantine" seems to have been deleted from the common vernacular. Interestingly, according to one local quarantine officer at YVR, "there has never been a case at the Vancouver International Airport where a full planeload of passengers has ever been 'held.'[22] The reasons for that are unclear, though a likely scenario readily presents itself.

• An alert flight attendant would report to the pilot that a particular passenger had generalized symptoms of flu, and was perhaps contagious. This is assuming that a flight attendant could, or would, spot a sick patient who may be most adept at controlling "shakes" and feigning sleep. The pilot would then forward that information to quarantine officials at his destination airport. On the tarmac, a quarantine nurse would become involved if deemed necessary. Once the other passengers had deplaned, the quarantine nurse would make a direct preliminary examination of the suspected sufferer. If suspicions were raised that the traveller may be suffering from an infectious disease, the victim would be directed or taken to a municipal hospital for a more thorough medical examination.

According to a spokesperson at YVR, only on occasion does a quarantine nurse actually enter an aircraft *before* other passengers have deplaned. When contagious disease is suspected, those passengers sitting "two rows in front and two rows behind,"[23] who may have unwittingly become contagious carriers, would also be identified and, if necessary, be prevented from proceeding through customs. The rest of the passengers would then be allowed to deplane. Those remaining on board would be advised of their rights and taken to the airport quarantine office. Where resistance is met from those who sat near the suffering passenger, airport security officers would be on hand to enforce detention.

• The obvious problem of this type of quarantine intervention is the identification and detention of particular healthy passengers who also might have had contact with an infected traveller. The recirculation of breathable air in a modern pressurized aircraft occurs swiftly throughout the whole plane. So strong is the air flow that it requires control from a panel above a passenger's seat. No doubt chemical air filters in these systems reduce the amount of airborne volatile organic compounds. The question is, do these filters restrict pathogens as minute as viruses, or do they merely distribute them throughout the whole aircraft? If they do not restrict viruses, as in the rooftop air filters suspected of spreading legionnaires' disease throughout Quebec City in 2012, the "two rows in front and two rows behind" detention rule for suspected aircraft passengers is completely fatuous.

In Montreal in 2007, the paucity of this regulation was tested. The *Montreal Star* carried the news that "all 28 passengers who sat near a man infected with a dangerous (multi-drug-resistant) strain of tuberculosis on Czech Airlines Flight 0104 from Prague to Montreal on May 24 have been identified."[24] At first glance, all seemed well in hand. However, Dr. H. Njoo, director of Canada's Public Health Agency added, "since we could not guarantee zero risk of transmission, we undertook certain measures."[25] Those measures included informing international health officials of all passengers on the flight, including those outside the five-row zone. Officials were urged to ask the potentially infected passengers to undergo tests for contagion. In Montreal, the Canadian passengers were contacted and asked to report to a toll-free line should they become ill. This self-reporting model undoubtedly saved Canadians money, but was it the best quarantine practice? In jurisdictions without ready phone access, such arm's-length self-reporting measures would be considered meagre.

In our economically conservative times, airport quarantine vigilance the world over seems wanting. With at least thirteen fatalities and sixty persons infected in China with the H7N9 bird flu, airports in New Zealand decided in 2013 not to step up airport screening. Has the rarity of airline-borne epidemics again nudged us into complacency? On April 22, 2013, the WHO reported that they "considered the risk of [an] international spread of the Avian Flu to be low."[26] Or has the world been beguiled by an ideological agenda that places public health ever lower in spending priorities? Cash-strapped Japan simply put up posters in its airports alerting Chinese travellers to seek medical help if required. In Singapore, Changi Airport planned only to distribute health leaflets to travellers arriving from China and the Middle East.

• • •

AT THE VANCOUVER INTERNATIONAL Airport, there is a quarantine office containing five quarantine officers (nurses) who work from 8:00 a.m. to midnight, seven days a week. From midnight to 8:00 a.m., when flights are largely suspended, there is *no* quarantine officer on-site, though a customs agent with some specialized training can be designated to act as a quarantine officer should such a necessity arise. After 4:00 p.m. daily, Vancouver International Airport or Calgary International also covers quarantine calls from smaller airports west of Manitoba.[27] East of Manitoba, such requests are directed to Toronto or Ottawa. Immediate two-way radio or telephone contact across the country to ambulance, security, or medically trained personnel seems to have replaced the "person on the ground" mentality of the quarantine stations of the past. Whether these modern adaptations of an old system are sufficient is a moot point.

According to one pilot, the Air Canada Handbook for the Airbus 320, a medium-range (5,400-kilometre) aircraft that can fly from Toronto or Vancouver to Cuba, Mexico, Hawaii, and the United States, contains no reference to quarantine in its table of contents. There is, however, guidance for the pilot regarding hijacking, bomb threats, disruptive passengers, and various mechanical or natural situations en route such as the eruption of a volcano.

One experienced Air Canada pilot informed me that the company does maintain a Medilink contact that patches inflight calls from the cockpit to appropriate medical officials on the ground in the case of a heart attack or death of a passenger during a flight. Flight attendants, he went on, *may* have reference to quarantine regulations and requirements on board. However, delays are costly and rescheduling is difficult and potentially libellous. In the reported pilot's years of experience on international flights, there are other more important issues than relaying suspected quarantine information to proper authorities. In tough economic times, when the bottom line for profit is miles flown, a meticulous application of Canada's quarantine regulations by air crew and cabin crew alike would not result in plaudits or promotions. Simply, it has become "something that is very much under the radar."[28]

So, with widespread global mobility fast replacing the old one-way direction of migration, new drug-resistant contagions have joined the international sojourn with relish. Unfortunately, those of us carrying them need attention, and with that come the ancient, furtive malevolencies of the human heart—indifference, arrogance, fear, brutality, and bigotry—all of which dogged the William Head Quarantine Station from its outset.

Beyond the airports, a new kind of quarantine station has evolved in Canada's larger urban centres. In Vancouver, for example, all medical wards in the city's larger hospitals have at least one room in each ward that is reserved as an isolation room. This is served by a team of health professionals known as the Infectious Disease Unit. At St. Paul's Hospital in Vancouver, the isolation rooms are negatively pressured such that internal air is prevented from escaping. When a sick person turns up at the emergency department of St. Paul's with the flu-like symptoms of a suspected contagion, the Infectious Diseases Unit is alerted. An emergency room physician orders a sample of blood, urine, or sputum be taken from the patient and sent to the Infectious Diseases Unit. There, confirmation of the suspected infectious agent such as the H1N1 flu virus is achieved through a test known as the polymerase chain reaction (PCR). Simply, the sample is machine-scanned for H1N1 or other virus genes. Once a virus is identified, the Infectious Disease Unit, in concert with emergency room physicians, establishes an appropriate antibiotic protocol for the patient, provided that the organism in question has not already become drug resistant.

Influenza with its rapid adaptive ability still remains a concern. In 2010, a mutant form of the H1N1 virus, H3N2, showed up at St. Paul's. In 2012, the virus caused America to suffer its worst outbreak in fifty years. In Vancouver, as elsewhere, research in therapies for drug-resistant pathogens is significant and ongoing. When HIV hit Vancouver in 1989 among gay men and drug users, sufferers began to show up at St. Paul's Hospital. As a Catholic hospital, St. Paul's had already established a long-standing association with the disenfranchised. In the days before a fully operative infectious disease unit was in place, HIV patients were initially isolated, not for reasons of contagion, but because they were simply seriously ill. Since that time the treatment of HIV/AIDS has changed considerably. No longer considered a disease with a certain death sentence, it is now treatable as an outpatient disease, because of the proven success of an antiretroviral "cocktail" established by Vancouver HIV/AIDS researcher Dr. Montaner. To serve that change, some infectious disease physicians at St. Paul's established a small outpatient practice to follow up on patients currently being treated for AIDS and other infectious diseases. It didn't always go so well.

Dr. Val Montessori commented on the Infectious Diseases Unit at St. Paul's:

When SARS arrived at St. Paul's in 1993–94, there was no plan because most physicians simply did not believe then that such a thing could happen. At the time, no one knew how the disease was spread . . . through the air (aerosol), or by other means such as direct contact. Hence, physicians with special training in infectious diseases were unsure whether to wear gowns, masks, or full, self-contained, oxygen-re-breathing suits. At the time, physicians requested the suits, but because their efficacy was unknown and their cost a premium, hospital administrators denied the request.[29]

Two cases of SARS *were* confirmed at St. Paul's Hospital in 2003–04. For want of something better, the patients were placed in isolated rooms in the Intensive Care Unit.

It didn't go so well, either, for the eradication of tuberculosis, and this disease currently remains the biggest concern for the Infectious Disease Unit at St. Paul's Hospital. According to Dr. Montessori, "many immigrants arrive in Vancouver with active tuberculosis and its incidence is also high among aboriginal peoples and drug users."[30] The disease is easily controlled with a six-month regimen of antibiotics. The difficulty is having the patients (especially intravenous drug users) take the pills regularly as required. To help facilitate this, St. Paul's Hospital has outreach nurses trained in tuberculosis treatment who visit the homes of active TB patients and assist in the agency of antibiotic therapy. If an infected patient leaves the Infectious Disease Unit against medical advice, a daily check of that person's known residence is made. Only rarely are police sent to retrieve the active patient.

The United Nations has reported that 81,000 new cases of multi-drug-resistant tuberculosis (MDR-TB) are being reported in Europe each year, with London being the most susceptible city.[31] Multi-drug-resistant tuberculosis does not seem to have found its way to Vancouver at this juncture, but when it does, the disenfranchised would be the first to be forced into further detention. Resistance seems natural.

• • •

WE ARE BACK TO where the story of the William Head Quarantine Station began. Canada, as well as the United States, has just emerged from a decade of paranoia that began with the terrorist attack on the World Trade Centre in New York on 9/11. In response, the right wing of American politics has demonstrably been pushed further to the right. In Canada, despite declining criminality, the Conservative government's Omnibus Crime Bill C-10 amended section 4(d) of the Corrections and Conditional Release Act, allowing for an increased use of force by prison guards against the incarcerated. Would such liberties be extended to guards securing new quarantine encampments? Some think so.

The question of how one ensures the balance between public safety and public liberty so as not to further suborn health officials with the socially conservative agenda of the political right has not changed. As such, quarantine remains now as much an issue of law as it once was at William Head.

The distinction between isolation and quarantine is at the heart of any regulations designed to curb the transmission of infectious diseases. Isolation is a control measure applied to people who are *already* ill. Quarantine is a measure applied to *healthy* people who are suspected of becoming ill in future and hence contagious. Often these individuals, as the William Head Quarantine Station's story has shown, greatly outnumber those who are actually ill. With pandemic influenzas once again in our midst, quarantine regulations must reflect this critical distinction. So how does one begin?

We begin by rejecting completely the idea that the best way to deal with a pandemic is to isolate the sick and contagious. Dr. Jenkins rejected the use of wholesale quarantine institutions in Alberta during the 1930s polio epidemic. Mayor Cope of Vancouver quarantined the whole city of Victoria to no avail after its 1892 epidemic of smallpox. Such wholesale use of quarantine is not only the stuff of fiction, as in Albert Camus's *The Plague*, it is also a policy that treads perilously close to ignoring time-honoured notions of civil liberty.

President George W. Bush not only wanted to re-establish large-scale quarantine institutions; in 2005, he argued that the office of the president should be granted increased special powers to bypass Congress. He wanted direct control, even if that meant his calling in the US Army. He said:

If we had an outbreak [of influenza] somewhere in the United States, do we not then quarantine that part of the country? And, who is best to be able to effect a quarantine? One option is the use of a military that's able to plan and move.

Congress needs to take a look at circumstances that may need to vest the capacity of the President with authority to move beyond the debate of the limits of Presidential power.[32]

The horror of Bush's plan was palpable. Did he mean to isolate all those healthy contagious individuals to special locations, such as a Super Bowl, where people would be herded and guarded by the military? Did he mean for the National Guard to stand at the gates of America's poorer towns and villages? That is *not* quarantine. In response, American pathologist Wendy Orent said, "If a health worker, drug addict, or teenager attempted to break out of that sort of large-scale quarantine facility, what would soldiers do? Shoot on sight?"[33] Bush's ill-conceived notions were quickly declared illegal. Calling in the troops has all the risks, and all the dread, as calling in un-informed and savage-minded members of the RCMP.

The central danger of President Bush's view is the concentration effect caused when suspected carriers are detained in a single location. Virus mutation and virulence in such an environment is increased as micro-organisms take advantage of a ready human food source. It has been said that the 1919 pandemic of Spanish influenza that killed millions began in the trenches of the Western Front, because the soldiers were "trapped" for a time in one huge "petri dish." As they moved to other parts of Europe and North America when hostilities ended, the virus simply moved with them, "becoming more virulent each time it encountered another concentrated, healthy population."[34] It wasn't enough that Canadians suffered sixty thousand war dead, fifty thousand more would perish of the Spanish Flu at home.

Unfortunately, George W. Bush was not alone in his singular conviction. Julie Gerberding, a director of the Centers for Disease Control and Prevention in America stated at the time that the military or National Guard might be summoned "to maintain civil order in the context of scarce resources or an overwhelming epidemic."[35] What that portends, one shudders to think.

• • •

THE ISSUE IS COMPLEX. Pandemics seem to be back, and with them are those contagious individuals who *do* need to be contained. Quarantine is necessary, even if it requires the short-term detention of more people than previously held in the quarantine institutions of the past. If the curtailment of infectious diseases is to remain a guiding principle, then modern quarantine regulations and those who carry them out must be seen to be without the influence of a right-wing social agenda. Like the judiciary, the politics of quarantine must be seen to be above the politics of favour or exclusion.

Without some sort of quarantine, we will have the pandemonium of those crazed by infectious disease. Quarantine law must allow officials to detect communicable diseases within our midst. They must be allowed to secure personal information in order to gather epidemiological information. Quarantine law must be strong enough to require citizens to comply with disease control measures such as examination and vaccination. Yet, such powers are at the very heart of individual freedoms in a liberal democracy. As Bennett has written, "Competing claims about the boundaries and meanings of public health law simply reflect competing claims about the boundaries for the legitimate exercise of political and administrative power."[36]

In that context, new quarantine legislation must contain certain assurances; the timelines of quarantine detention must be thoroughly explained. Those detained must have assurance that they will be properly cared for with sufficient food, clothing, and shelter. Quarantine officials must have training in human ethics and must also be seen to comply with rules governing human dignity.

The William Head Quarantine Station was dogged by the exigencies of human malevolence from its very beginnings. But it also had its time of success, hard won by those humanitarians who would not settle for anything less. As the reality of pandemic again enters our consciousness, changing public health policies on quarantine must be seen to clearly embrace human rights *and* treatment.

That issue lies at the heart of this book. In the context of these larger concerns, vaccination seems to be the least of our worries and still remains our best medicine.

AFTERWORD // MEMORIAL PLAQUES AT WILLIAM HEAD

I am not yet born; forgive me for the sins
that in me, the world shall commit.

—Louis MacNeice, "Prayer Before Birth"[1]

Sadly, there is not much left of the forty-two buildings that once comprised the William Head Quarantine Station. The first-class hospital, first-class detention house, second-class hospital, and isolation houses, not to mention the Chinese and Japanese detention units, are all gone. So, too, are the physicians' residences, the warden's and guards' houses, staff residences, laboratory, laundry, and wharf. Most of the original clapboard structures, built when the station was first opened in 1893, are gone, and most of the fumigation equipment such as the huge steel sterilizing retorts, railway tracks, and disinfection carts have simply vanished.

However, the federal penitentiary service, since it acquired the site for a minimum-security prison in 1958, has generally been a good custodian. Some significant buildings do remain, and the service has made an honest attempt to have others moved and restored. The schoolhouse and chapel building is still there, restored and gleaming in its 1920s red-brick facade, as is the original administration building. The brick exteriors of the fumigation building, disinfection-storage building, and bathhouse remain, as do the footings of foghorns and navigation lights at the seaward end of the peninsula. Original plans and photographs remain in abundance. The old quarantine station cemetery is still tended, its crosses marking the final place of those who could not be cured of the contagion they carried.

Kim Rempel, prison librarian, has created a special historic photographic exhibition of the William Head Quarantine Station during its best years for current inmates, visitors, and staff. He feels, as I and others do, that memorial plaques and perhaps information kiosks should be strategically placed throughout the site to commemorate those of the Chinese Labour Corps and others who could not be cured of their contagion. Save for a complete rededication and reconstruction of the William Head Quarantine Station as a National Historic Site, as has occurred at Grosse Île, Quebec, such plaques are the very least we can do to remind ourselves of the role this once-proud medical complex played in our history.

The William Head Quarantine Station was once a symbol on the grandest scale. Its significance goes far beyond the west coast's struggle against infectious disease. It made heroes of the men and women who acted with perseverance and compassion, enabling, finally, a permanent link with those around the Pacific Rim. Its stories dramatically revealed the continuing need for humane quarantine legislation in order to protect those threatened by contagion and to safeguard individuals against the prevailing prejudices and indifferences of the state.

ACKNOWLEDGEMENTS

This book would not have been written without the help and encouragement of Margaret Roper, president (2001–11) and curator of the Metchosin School Museum Society. Her enthusiasm for the story of the William Head Quarantine Station inspired me to the very end. When I was racked with frustration over an incomplete trail of information, Margaret, ever the sleuth, often uncovered a lead that opened the way ahead. Jennifer Kitching, reference librarian at the British Columbia Legislative Library, provided me with a bibliography of early BC newspapers. Andrew Martin and Kate Russell, special collections librarians at the Vancouver Public Library, nurtured me through the complexities of Ottawa's Sessional Papers and unearthed early photographs. UBC special collections archivist Sarah Romkey found early shipping information. Anna Krangle-Long and Rebecca Slaven of the Bio-Medical Library at the University of British Columbia directed me to early epidemiological journals, and Lisa Glandt, librarian at the Vancouver Maritime Museum, provided photographs of the more famous ships that were connected with the William Head Quarantine Station. Archivist Sarah Rather at the City of Victoria Archives also helped immensely, as did Chantal Jacques, assistant warden at the William Head Penitentiary, and Kim Rempel, librarian at that facility. Photographers Sarah Pugh and researcher Sofia Dönnecke were wonderful. These custodians of our cultural heritage are invaluable.

I would especially like to thank my friend and colleague John Gellard for editing an early draft. His attention to grammar and style helped immensely. John Pearce also gave much encouragement. Dr. Brian G. Sparkes of Panmed International provided immunological background. Dr. Val Montessori of the Division of Infectious Diseases at St. Paul's Hospital, Vancouver, told me of its current measures in quarantine medicine. I was fortunate to find several people, now in their nineties, who worked at the quarantine station during its early years. Interviewing Beth Harmon (née Ellwood) and Joan Watkins (née Pears) was a sheer joy. Both knew each other in the 1930s, and their stories validated other tales of life at William Head during its best years. Doug Corbett and Mike Lee were children at the station during the Depression. Faith Walton Lee knew everyone at the station school in the 1930s, and gladly reminisced.

Conversations with Diana Turner (née Jenkins), daughter of Dr. R.B. Jenkins, chief medical officer at the station, were a delight. She fleshed out the work of her father, in the 1940s and 1950s, only hinted at in documents. Her husband, Maurice Turner, "Migs," a naval lieutenant during the Second World War, added much about the effect of the war years on life at William Head. The unpublished reminiscences of Violet Rainey (née Rhode) and Marjorie Rhode spoke eloquently of life at William Head in the 1920s. Long-time cycling friends Lynn and Donnamae Wilson of Sidney, BC, welcomed me and my enthusiasms in my seemingly endless visits to numerous archives and museums on Vancouver Island. Friend, gentleman-adventurer, and long-distance cyclist Hank Westervelt shared my love of history. Our ongoing discussions about some truly brilliant writers and their ability to bring the past to life inspired me to keep going.

ENDNOTES

Chapter 1

1. Emma Lazarus, as quoted in Ann Novotny, *Strangers at the Door: Ellis Island, Castle Garden, and the Great Immigration to America* (Riverside, Connecticut: Chatham Press, 1971), p. 143. The biggest difference between the Ellis Island Quarantine and Immigration Station in New York and Canadian stations in, say, Halifax or Grosse Île, Quebec is that Ellis Island was in essence a clearing station for screening more than just the entry of infectious diseases to American shores. At Ellis Island, would-be new Americans were given an English language test (some forty words), an I.Q. test, a means test (indigent immigrants who would cost America money were not allowed), and a strict moral screening (prostitutes and criminals were disbarred). In Canada, issues beyond preventing the entrance of immigrants on social and intellectual grounds lay with the customs agents. Only in the 1950s, when the quarantine station at William Head had very few quarantine detentions, did medical officials take over the task of customs agents . . . but only for a very short time.

President John F. Kennedy was the great-grandson of an Irish immigrant, and never forgot the powerlessness of millions of indigent Irish who arrived in New York in the latter half of the nineteenth century. As a young congressman, Kennedy sponsored the Displaced Persons Act in 1948. In presenting the bill, Kennedy thought that Lazarus's poem should be amended to read "Give me your tired, your poor . . . as long as they come from Northern Europe, are not too tired, or too poor, or slightly ill, never stole a loaf of bread, never joined any questionable organization, and can document their activities for the past two years."

2. Howard Markel, *Quarantine: Jewish Immigrants in New York City during the Epidemic of 1892* (Baltimore: Johns Hopkins University Press, 1997), 13.

3. F. Gensini, M. Yacoub, and A. Conti, "The Concept of Quarantine in History: From Plague to SARS," *Journal of Infection*, no. 49 (2004), 257.

4. J.H. Kilwein. "Some Historical Comments on Quarantine: Part 1," *Journal of Clinical Pharmacy and Therapeutics* 20 (1995), 185.

5. F. Gensini, et al., "The Concept of Quarantine in History," 258.

6. Ernest Gilman, "The Art of Medicine," *The Lancet* 373 (June 2009), 2018.

7. Ibid., 2019.

8. J.H. Kilwein, "Some Historical Comments on Quarantine," 186. In Britain, the dying, if they had the means or were of the right class, were also buried, only to be exhumed

and the wooden coffins burned as ordinary firewood by the poor. See also George Alfred Walker, *Burial Ground Incendiarism* (London: Longman & Co., 1845), 10.

9. Ibid., 28.

10. J.H. Kilwein, "Some Historical Comments of Quarantine: Part 2," *Journal of Clinical Pharmacy and Therapeutics* 20 (1995), 250.

11. Ibid.

12. Krista Maglen, "Politics of Quarantine in the 19th Century," *Journal of the American Medical Association* no. 21 (December 2003), 2873.

13. David Heymann, *Model Operational Guidelines for Disease Exposure Control* (Washington, D.C.: Centre for Strategic and International Studies Homeland Security Program, 2005), 9. http://csis.org/files/media/csis/pubs/051102_dec_guidelines.pdf.

14. Howard Markel, *Quarantine: Jewish Immigrants in New York City*, 155.

15. Ibid., 72.

16. Howard Markel, *When Germs Travel* (New York: Pantheon Books, 2004), 25.

17. Paul Edelson, "Quarantine and Social Inequity," *Journal of the American Medical Association* 290, no. 21 (December 2003), 2874.

18. David Heymann, *Model Operational Guidelines for Disease Exposure Control*, 11.

19. John Heagerty, *Four Centuries of Medical History in Canada*, Vol. 1 (Toronto: MacMillan, 1928), 177.

20. Edgar Wickberg, ed., *From China to Canada: A History of Chinese Communities in Canada* (Toronto: McClelland & Stewart, 1988), 66.

21. Ibid., 67.

22. Besides the truly poor, tuberculosis also spread among those who exhibited the sexually promiscuous lifestyle of the new bohemians, and became associated with the free spirits, artists, dilettantes, thieves, and other "flower children" of the period. Dostoevsky, Goethe, Keats, Chopin, Stravinsky, Kafka, Modigliani, the Bronte sisters and Robert Louis Stevenson all died from tuberculosis, and so, besides being deadly, it gained somewhat of a romantic and seductive cachet. Mimi, the pale-faced heroine of Puccini's La Boheme, dies exhausted at the end of the story of unrequited love and tuberculosis, a classic victim of the "white plague."

23. Paul Farmer, *Pathologies of Power* (Berkeley: University of California Press, 2003), 130.

24. Ibid., 128.

25. Ibid., 184.

26. Ibid., 184.

27. Helena Hansen and Nora Groce, "Human Immunodeficiency Virus and Quarantine in Cuba," *Journal of the American Medical Association* 290, no. 21 (December 2003), 2875.

Chapter 2

1. Peter Puget, "Log of the Discovery, May 7–June 11, 1792," *Pacific Northwest Quarterly* 30, no. 2 (April 1939), 229–30.

2. *The British Colonist*, March 26, 1862, 3. See also March 18, 1862.

3. Ibid., 3.

4. Douglas Hamilton, "The Great Pox," *Rain Coast Chronicles*, no. 17 (1996), 32.

5. Ibid., 35.

6. *The British Colonist,* June 16, 1862, 3.

7. *The British Colonist,* July 7, 1862, 3.

8. *The British Colonist,* August 18, 1862, 3.

9. Richard Mackie, *The Wilderness Profound* (Victoria: SoNoNis Press, 1995), 30.

10. Letter from President of Board of Health to Provincial Secretary, July 2, 1872. archives.leg.bc./EPLlibraries.leg_arc/document/ID 534021082.

11. Ibid.

12. Ibid.

13. Letter from Dr. Matthews to City of Victoria Board of Health, June 2, 1872. archives.leg.bc./EPL libraries.leg_arc/document/ID/534021082.

14. *The British Colonist,* June 15, 1872, 3.

15. Ibid., 3.

16. *The British Colonist,* June 14, 1872, 3.

17. This is confirmed in two letters from the Board of Health, one dated June 24 from W.B. Matthews to Captain Williams, and another dated June 28 from Mr. Leigh (Secretary to Board of Health) to H.G. Williams, granting him permission to get water from Esquimalt Lagoon. At archives.leg.bc/EPL libraries.leg._arc/document/ID/5340211082.

18. Janis Ringuette, *Beacon Hill Park History 1842–2009,* www.beaconhillparkhistory.org.

19. *The British Colonist,* June 19, 1872, 3.

20. *The British Colonist,* June 15, 1872, 3.

21. *The British Colonist,* June 16, 1872, 3.

22. *The British Colonist,* June 15, 1872, 3.

23. *The British Colonist,* June 17, 1872, 5.

24. *The British Colonist,* June 15, 1872, 3.

25. *The British Colonist,* June 19, 1872, 3.

26. *The British Colonist,* June 18, 1872, 3.

27. Ibid.

28. Ibid.

29. Ibid.

30. Ibid.

31. Ibid.

32. *The British Colonist,* June 20, 1872, 3.

33. Ibid.

34. *The British Colonist,* June 18, 1872, 3.

35. Letter from Peter Eddy to the Victoria Board of Health, June 24, 1872. At archives.leg.bc/EPLlibraries.leg_arc/document/ID/5340211082.

36. Ibid.

37. Ibid.

38. *The British Colonist,* June 22, 1872, 3.

39. *The British Colonist,* June 25, 1873, 3.

40. Ibid.

41. Ibid.

42. The Hon. Justice Gray, *The Quarantine Claims, Prince Alfred, June 1872* (Victoria, BC: Victoria Standard Printers, December 1873).

43. Ibid., 4.

44. The Hon. Justice Gray, *The Quarantine Claims, Prince Alfred, June 1872* (Victoria, BC: Victoria Standard Printers, December 1873), 8.

45. Ibid.

46. Ibid.

47. Ibid., 9

48. Ibid., 9

49. Ibid., 10.

50. The Hon. Justice Gray, *The Quarantine Claims*, December 1873, 101.

51. Ibid.

52. *Victoria Daily Colonist*, July 11, 1884, 2.

53. Memorandum for Dr. Bain, Quarantine Station, William Head, October 17, 1938, 1. In miscellaneous file, British Columbia Legislative Library, Parliament Buildings, Victoria, BC.

54. *Victoria Daily Colonist*, September 19, 1884, 3.

55. Bart Armstrong, "Quarantined in Name Only: The Albert Head Story," *The Islander*, June 17, 1984, 4.

56. *The British Colonist,* June 12, 1872, 3.

Chapter 3

1. Margaret Atwoood, "Further Arrivals," in Leuba Bailey, ed., *The Immigrant Experience* (Toronto: MacMillan of Canada, 1975), 24.

2. *Victoria Daily Colonist*, September 16, 1892, 6.

3. Ibid.

4. Vertical file. British Columbia Pioneer Physicians, Woodward Medical Library Rare Books Division, University of British Columbia. Under *Jones, William Macnaughton*, uncatalogued, 2012.

5. Ibid.

6. Gerry Ferguson, "Control of the Insane in British Columbia, 1849–78," in John McLaren, Robert Menzies, Dorothy E. Chunn, eds., *Regulating Lives: Historical Essays on the State, Society, the Individual, and the Law* (Vancouver: UBC Press, 2002), 85.

7. Sessional Papers, no. 10A (Ottawa, 1886), 178.

8. *Victoria Daily Colonist*, October 20, 1892, 3.

9. Norman Hacking and William Kaye Lamb, *The Princess Story* (Vancouver: Mitchell Press Ltd., 1974), 120.

10. Ibid., 121.

11. Sessional Papers, no. 6A (Ottawa, 1891), 24.

12. Ibid.

13. Ibid.

14. Ibid.

15. Ibid, 25.

16. *Victoria Daily Colonist*, October 20, 1892, 3.

17. Sessional Papers, vol. 26, no. 5 (Ottawa, 1893), 18.

18. *Victoria Daily Colonist*, October 20, 1892, 3.

19. *Victoria Daily Colonist*, July 8, 1892, 5.

20. Ibid.

21. Theodore F. Rose, *From Shaman to Modern Medicine: A Century of the Healing Arts in British Columbia* (Vancouver: Mitchell Press, 1972), 30.

22. *Victoria Daily Colonist*, July 16, 1892, 4.

23. Ibid.

24. *Victoria Daily Colonist*, July 12, 1892, 3.

25. T.F. Rose, *From Shaman to Modern Medicine*, 131

26. *Vancouver Daily News-Advertiser*, July 13, 1892, 3.

27. *Victoria Daily Colonist*, July 13, 1892, 4.

28. Ibid.

29. Ibid.

30. Ibid.

31. Hacking and Lamb, *The Princess Story*, 106.

32. *Victoria Daily Colonist*, July 15, 1892, 4.

33. *Victoria Daily Colonist*, July 21, 1892, 3.

34. Hacking and Lamb, *The Princess Story*, 123.

35. Ibid.

36. *Victoria Daily Colonist*, July 29, 1892, 6.

37. See Patricia Johnson, "McCreight and the Bench," *British Columbia Historical Quarterly* 13, no. 3 (July 1948), 222. Also, the text of Justice McCreight's judgement as reported in the *Vancouver Daily News-Advertiser*, July 23, 1892, 4.

38. *Vancouver Daily News-Advertiser*, July 23, 1892, 4.

39. That figure (50 cases) was based on the testimony of Dr. Morrison, Victoria Health Officer. See *Victoria Daily Colonist*, July 29, 1892, 6.

40. Ibid.

41. Ibid.

42. Ibid.

43. Ibid.

44. Ibid.

45. *Victoria Daily Colonist*, July 26, 1892, 4.

46. *Victoria Daily Colonist*, July 23, 1892, 4.

47. Ibid.

48. *Victoria Daily Colonist*, July 13, 1892, 4.

49. *Victoria Daily Colonist*, July 15, 1892, 3.

50. *Victoria Daily Colonist*, July 26, 1892, 4.

51. *Victoria Daily Colonist*, July 27, 1892, 4.

52. Ibid.

53. Hacking and Lamb, *The Princess Story*, 123.

54. Alexander St. Paul Butler, "Short History of William Head," unpublished manuscript,

55. Metchosin School Museum, Metchosin, BC, 25.

Chapter 4

1. David Helwig, "One Step from an Old Dance," In *An Anthology of Canadian Literature in English* (Toronto: University of Toronto Press, 1973), 213.

2. *Victoria Daily Colonist*, March 13, 1893, 3.

3. Ibid.

4. Ibid.

5. Ibid.

6. *Victoria Daily Colonist*, September 17, 1892, 4.

7. *Victoria Daily Colonist*, July 21, 1892, 3.

8. Ibid.

9. Ibid.

10. Ibid.

11. *Victoria Daily Colonist*, July 28, 1892, 6.

12. Ibid.

13. *Victoria Daily Colonist*, July 30, 1892, 5.

14. Ibid.

15. Correspondence of Dr. Huntley to Dr. J.C. Davie, August 10, 1892, in Sessional Papers, vol. 56 (Victoria, BC: British Columbia Legislature, 1892), 276.

16. Ibid., 276.

17. Ibid., 279.

18. *Victoria Daily Colonist*, July 28, 1892, 6.

19. "Report on the Commission to Inquire into the Late Epidemic Outbreak of Small-pox in the Province of British Columbia, under Order in Council, Dated the 6th October, 1892," in Sessional Papers 6-3, British Columbia Public Accounts, July 1891–June 1892 (Victoria, BC: Queens Printer), 507.

20. *Victoria Daily Colonist*, October 29, 1892, 3.

21. Ibid.

22. "Report on the Commission to Inquire into the Late Epidemic Outbreak of Smallpox in the Province of British Columbia," 508.

23. *Victoria Daily Colonist*, October 21, 1892, 3.

24. Ibid.

25. Ibid.

26. Ibid. Yet a day earlier, the *Colonist* reported that Dr. Hall and Dr. Leigh visited the child "the next day," which would be Thursday, and both went to Dr. Milne's office to make a report. On Saturday, Dr. Crompton, another Victoria health officer, confirmed that the boy had smallpox. What or who to believe? *Victoria Daily Colonist*, October 20, 1892, 3.

27. *Victoria Daily Colonist*, October 21, 1892, 3.

28. "Report on the Commission to Inquire into the Late Epidemic Outbreak of Smallpox in the Province of British Columbia," 510.

29. *Victoria Daily Colonist*, October 20, 1892, 3.

30. "Report on the Commission to Inquire into the Late Epidemic Outbreak of Smallpox," 510.

31. *Victoria Daily Colonist*, October 20, 1892, 3.

32. *Victoria Daily Colonist*, December 15, 1892, 5.

33. "Report on the Commission to Inquire into the Late Epidemic Outbreak of Smallpox," 510.

34. Mr. Huntley confirmed this date within his letter to the Provincial Medical Officer. British Columbia Sessional Papers, vol. 56, 278.

35. "Report on the Commission to Inquire into the Late Epidemic Outbreak of Smallpox," 510.

36. Ibid.

37. Ibid.

38. Ibid., 517.

39. *Victoria Daily Colonist*, January 7, 1893, 6.

40. Ibid.

41. Ibid.

42. Ibid.

43. Ibid.

44. Sessional Papers, no. 7A (Ottawa, 1893), 18.

45. *Victoria Daily Colonist*, March 3, 1893, 3.

Chapter 5

1. *Victoria Daily Colonist*, July 29, 1892, 6.

2. Ibid.

3. Irwin Shermin, *Twelve Diseases that Shook the World* (Washington, D.C.: ASM Press, 2007), 40.

4. Paul de Kruif, *Microbe Hunters* (New York: Harcourt Brace, 1926), 125.

5. Irwin Shermin, *Twelve Diseases*, 33.

6. *Victoria Daily Colonist*, September 13, 1892, 3.

7. Ibid.

8. *Victoria Daily Colonist*, September 1, 1893, 8.

9. Ibid.

10. Ibid.

11. Ibid.

12. Ibid.

13. Ibid.

14. Ibid.

15. Ibid.

16. Ibid.

17. Ibid.

18. Ibid.

19. The *Victoria Daily Colonist*, August 29, 1893, 5.

20. The *Victoria Daily Colonist*, May 27, 1893, 6.

21. Sessional Papers vol. 28, no.5 (Ottawa, 1895), 27-28.

22. Ibid., 27.

23. Ibid., 28.

24. Vertical file. Uncatalogued. Woodward Medical Library, Rare Books Division. University of British Columbia. *Profile of BC Medical Pioneers*

25. *Victoria Daily Colonist*, October 26, 1896, 5.

26. *Victoria Daily Colonist*, January 4, 1897, 3.

27. *Victoria Daily Colonist*, September 15, 1900, 7.

28. Ibid.

29. Ibid.

30. Ibid.
31. Ibid.
32. Ibid.
33. Ibid.
34. *Victoria Daily Colonist*, February 5, 1902, 4.
35. Ibid.
36. *Victoria Daily Colonist*, May 3, 1903, 10.
37. *Victoria Daily Colonist*, February 5, 1902, 4.

Chapter 6

1. *Victoria Daily Colonist*, May 28, 1907, 10.
2. Sessional Papers, vol. 32, no. 10 (Ottawa, 1897), 58.
3. *Victoria Daily Colonist*, February 4, 1908, 10.
4. Sessional Papers, vol. 32, no. 10 (Ottawa, 1897), 58.
5. First-class menu from *Empress of India*, January 1, 1917.
6. Robert Turner, *The Pacific Empresses* (Victoria: Sono Nis Press, 1981), 171.
7. *Victoria Daily Colonist*, April 30, 1897, 7.
8. Robert D. Turner, *The Pacific Empresses*, 40.

Chapter 7

1. *Victoria Daily Colonist*, January 5, 1893, 4.
2. Correspondence with Minister of Agriculture, December 31, 1902. Ottawa: National Archives of Canada.
3. *Victoria Daily Colonist*, January 16, 1901, 6.
4. *Victoria Daily Colonist*, February 15, 1902, 5.
5. Correspondence with Dr. Montizambert, Director-General of Public Health, April 1, 1909. National Archives of Canada.
6. Correspondence to Minister of Agriculture from A. T. Watt, March 31, 1912. Sessional Papers, British Columbia Legislature. Group 12–15, Volume XLVII, No. 8, 1913, 98.
7. *Victoria Daily Times*, July 9, 1913, 18.
8. Ibid., 98.
9. Dr. A.T. Watt, correspondence to the Minister of Agriculture, Ottawa, March 31, 1913, in Canada Department of Public Health, Reports on the Division of Quarantine, 1897-1-1956. BC Archives, B-8643, GR 2005.
10. Sessional Papers, British Columbia Legislature. Group 12 -15, Volume XLVII, No.8, 1913, 98.
11. *Vancouver Sun*, April 2, 1913, 1.
12. *Victoria Daily Colonist*, April 1, 1913, 4.
13. *Victoria Daily Colonist*, April 9, 1913, 4.
14. Ibid.
15. *Vancouver Sun*, June 2, 1913, 1.
16. *Victoria Daily Times*, May 23, 1913, 20.
17. Ibid., 20.
18. Ibid., 20.

19. *Victoria Daily Times*, May 23, 1913, 20.

20. *Victoria Daily Times*, June 6, 1913, 16.

21. *Victoria Daily Times*, June 6, 1913, 16.

22. Ibid.

23. *Victoria Daily Times*, May 23, 1913, 20.

24. *Victoria Daily Times*, May 30, 1913, 23.

25. Ibid.

26. Ibid.

27. Ibid., 1.

28. Edward Laxton, *The Famine Ships: The Irish Exodus to America* (London: Bloomsbury, 1996), 39. Built in 1763 for 150 passengers, the *Elizabeth and Sarah* was worn out long before her work as a famine ship. When she set out from Killala, County Mayo in 1847, she carried nearly 300 passengers. When she arrived in Quebec, 21 had died, but 250 were seriously ill.

29. Correspondence from R.S. Kinney to Hon. Martin Burrell, Minister of Agriculture, April 19, 1913. Quoted in Linda M. Ambrose, "Quarantine in Question: The 1913 Investigation at William Head," *Canadian Bulletin of Medical History* 22, no.1 (2005). I am indebted to Dr. Ambrose's excellent paper on Dr. Watt's suicide while under investigation in 1913. It sets out eloquently and succinctly the conflicting class, racial, and political questions that arose from the incident.

30. *Victoria Daily Times*, June 6, 1913, 16.

31. Ibid.

32. Ibid.

33. Ibid.

34. Ibid.

35. *Victoria Daily Times*, May 30, 1913, 1.

36. Ibid.

37. Ibid., 3.

38. *Vancouver Sun*, June 2, 1913, 1.

39. Ibid., 18.

40. Ibid., 22.

41. Ibid., 150.

42. Linda Ambrose, "Quarantine in Question," 153. This is a wonderful piece of scholarly digging. The verses are two and four from part 79 of *In Memoriam*.

43. *Victoria Daily Times*, July 28, 1913, 1.

44. *Vancouver Sun*, July 29, 1913, 1.

45. *Victoria Daily Times*, July 28, 1913, 1.

46. *Victoria Daily Times*, July 30, 1913, 4.

47. *Victoria Daily Times*, September 5, 1913, 4.

Chapter 8

1. Earle Birney, "Anglosaxon Street," in *The Immigrant Experience*, Leuba Bailey, ed. (Toronto: MacMillan of Canada, 1975), 59.

2. J. Robert Davison, "The Chinese at William Head, A Photograph Album," *British Columbia Historical News,* 16, no. 4 (1983), 19.

3. Cliff Chandler, "Chinese Labour Camps at William Head Quarantine Station, 1917–1920," *Victoria Historical Society Publication,* no. 17 (Autumn 2008), 2.

4. Nancy de Bertrand Lugrin, "10,000 Coolies and a Lost Little Girl," *Victoria Sunday Times Magazine,* August 11, 1951, 3.

5. Ibid.

6. Cliff Chandler, "Chinese Labour Camps at William Head," 2.

7. Lisa Smedman, "Coolie Express," *Vancouver Courier,* June, 26, 2009, 1.

8. Ibid., 3

9. Ibid.

10. Ibid. 2, as cited from an unnamed source.

11. Marion Helgesen, *Footnotes: Pioneer Families of the Metchosin District, 1851–1900* (Metchosin, BC: Metchosin School Museum Society, 1983), 262.

12. Nancy de Bertrand Lugrin, "10,000 Coolies," 3.

13. Ibid.

14. Ibid.

15. J. Robert Davison, "The Chinese at William Head," 19.

16. Lisa Smedman, "Coolie Express," 4.

17. Cliff Chandler, "Chinese Labour Camps at William Head," 3.

18. *The Islander,* December 6, 1981, 10.

19. Ibid.

20. Lisa Smedman, 5.

21. Cliff Chandler, "Chinese Labour Camps at William Head," 3.

22. Ibib., 43.

23. Television interview with Ray Gray, son of Percy Gray, on The Pepper Patch, Victoria Community Television, March 1989.

24. J. Robert Davison, "The Chinese at William Head," 19.

25. Ibid., 20.

26. *Times Colonist,* June 25, 2009, 4.

27. Ibid.

28. Ibid.

29. *Daily Province,* March 29, 1920, 3.

30. From the menu of the William Head Repatriation Supper. Unclassified. The William Head collection. Metchosin School Museum. n.d.

31. *The Oxford Companion to Canadian History,* Gerald Hallowell, ed. (Oxford University Press: Don Mills, Ontario, 2004), 128.

32. Chris Yorath, *A Measure of Value: The Story of D'Arcy Island* (Victoria: Touchwood Editions, 2000), p. 59.

33. Renisa Mawani, "'The Island of the Unclean': Race, Colonialism and 'Chinese Leprosy' in British Columbia, 1891–1924, *Law, Social Justice and Global Development,* no.1 (2003), 9, http://www2.warwick.ac.uk/fac/soc/law/elj/lgd/2003_1/mawani/.

34. Ibid.

35. *Victoria Daily Colonist,* July 5, 1899, 3.

36. *Victoria Daily Colonist,* September 2, 1879, 10.

37. Ilma Salazar Gourley, "D'Arcy Island, 1891–1907," *British Columbia Historical News* 18, no. 3 (1985), 8.

38. Ibid., 7.

39. Renisa Mawani, "The Island of the Unclean," 11.

40. Ibid., 10.

41. Ibid.

42. Ibid.

43. Chris Yorath, *A Measure of Value*, 41–48.

44. *Victoria Daily Colonist*, September 2, 1979, 10.

45. Ilma Salazar Gourley, "D'Arcy Island, 1891–1907," 8.

46. Renisa Mawani, "The Island of the Unclean," 12.

47. Ilma Salazar Gourley, "D'Arcy Island, 1891–1907," 8.

48. Renisa Mawani, "The Island of the Unclean," 12.

49. Ibid.

50. *Victoria Daily Colonist*, September 2, 1979, 10.

51. Ibid., 12.

52. Guenther Krueger, "The Lepers of Bentinck," *The Beaver* 69, no. 3 (June/July 1989), 60.

53. Ibid.

54. Ibid.

55. Guenther Krueger, unpublished interview with Dr. Jenkins, June 18, 1988.

56. *Victoria Daily Colonist*, June 10, 1965, 4.

57. Guenther Krueger interview with Dr. Jenkins, July 18, 1988.

58. Ibid., 4.

59. *Victoria Daily Colonist*, January 5, 1952, 5.

60. *Victoria Daily Colonist*, January 22, 1954, 1.

61. Cy Young, "Lepers' Island," *MacLean's Magazine*, May 1, 1948, 24.

62. Guenther Kreuger, "The Lepers of Bentinck," 65.

63. *Times Colonist*, September 2, 1979, 10.

Chapter 9

1. Slated somewhere between February 2 and March 9 each year, depending upon the date of Easter. Shrove Tuesday was a popular Christian day of feasting, games, rowdiness, and mischief the day before Ash Wednesday, the onset of the period of fasting called Lent. It was called Pancake Tuesday or Pancake Day in Britain and was celebrated for many centuries. It became a school holiday in the nineteenth century. "Shroving," or Lent Crocking, was the practice in Exmoor and the West Country where children with blackened faces would creep into a neighbour's house the evening of Pancake Tuesday and throw broken crockery over the floor and run away. The verb is derived from "shriving," or "to shrive," meaning to confess (one's sins) before Lent. This rhyme, and many others like it, was common among school children all over England before WWII. In Iona and Peter Opie, *The Lore and Language of School Children* (London: Oxford University Press, 1959), 239.

2. Ibid.

3. Letter of reference to Secretary, Wm. Head station school, from E.B. Paul, Supt. of Schools, Victoria, October 18, 1909.

4. Interview with Joan Watkins (née Pears), March 17, 2010. Joan, who was ninety-four at the time of our interview, pioneered with her parents in Metchosin, near the quarantine station. She knew many of the children who lived at the station, befriended some, and associated with many.

5. Unpublished reminiscences of the quarantine station, 1915–28, by Violet E. Rainey, Metchosin School Museum, 1.

6. Ibid.

7. A personal interview with Michael Lee, September 8, 2010. At 85, Michael still remembered much of his life at the William Head Quarantine Station. He was born there, educated there, worked there, and retired there as a deckhand on the station's launches in 1958 and then as a prison guard at the William Head Penitentiary, in 1974.

8. Private correspondence with Douglas Corbett, October 13, 2010.

9. Violet Rainey, reminiscences of William Head Quarantine Station, 3.

10. Ibid.

11. Interview with Faith Walton (née Lee), September 28, 2010, in Sidney, British Columbia. Faith was 91 at the time and had lived on the Station until the mid-1930s when she left for high school in Victoria.

12. Sieka Boye, "An interview with Leland Windreich," *Dance Collection Danse* (March 2010), 20.

13. Ibid., 3.

14. Ibid., 4.

15. Violet Rainey, reminiscences of William Head Quarantine Station.

16. Interview with Faith Walton, September 28, 2010.

17. Ibid.

18. Ibid.

19. *Victoria Daily Colonist*, February 19, 1950, Sunday magazine edition, 1.

20. As told to Maurice Turner, husband of Diana Jenkins, in an interview on April 8, 2010.

21. Gordon Newell, "Maritime Events of 1929–1930," in H.W. McCurdy, *Marine History of the Pacific Northwest* (Seattle: Superior, 1966), 404.

22. Interview with Beth Harmon (Ellwood), daughter of Alexander Ellwood who ran the Metchosin General Store from 1924–47, February 15, 2010. Beth was ninety at the time of the interview.

23. Interview with Diana Jenkins, April 8, 2010.

24. Interview with Elizabeth Harmon (nee Ellwood), February 15, 2010.

25. Interview with Michael Lee, September 8, 2010.

26. Interview with Joan Watkins (née Pears), of Metchosin, March 17, 2010.

27. Ibid.

28. Ibid.

29. Ibid.

30. Andrew St. Paul Butler, unpublished manuscript on the history of William Head, 54.

31. "A conversation with Mrs. Marjorie Rhode, 1931–1960," Metchosin School Museum, n.d.

32. Correspondence with Maurice "Migs" Turner, April 8, 2010.

33. Interview with Mike Lee, September 8, 2010.

34. All of the material for this more social history of life at the William Head Quarantine Station came from direct interviews and transcripts of previous correspondences with half a dozen people who lived at the station from the 1920s through to its demise in 1958. Mike Lee died three weeks after my interview with him in Kelowna, BC, on October 2, 2010.

35. Interview with Mike Lee, September 8, 2010.

Chapter 10

1. *Vancouver Province*, June 4, 1956, 6. See also Andrew St. Paul Butler, 50.

2. Dr. F. Montizambert, "The Story of 54 Years' Quarantine Service from 1866 to 1920," *The Canadian Medical Association Journal* 16, no. 3 (March 1926), 318.

3. *Daily Province*, March 1, 1925, 10.

4. Ibid.

5. Ibid.

6. Ibid.

7. Ibid.

8. Ibid.

9. Ibid.

10. Ibid.

11. Chester Brown, Annual Report to Ottawa, 1927/1928, 2.

12. Dr. C. Brown, Report to the Deputy Minister of Health. Sessional Papers, Public Health Canada, Appendix No. 1, (Ottawa, 1926), 101.

13. Ibid., 1.

14. Ibid., 1.

15. Government of Canada Annual Departmental Reports, 1937–38, Vol. 3, Dept. of Pensions and National Health, 126.

16. Chester Brown, Annual Report to Ottawa. In letter to Dr. J.D. Page, Chief Quarantine Division, Department of Pensions and National Health, April 30, 1929, 1.

17. Ibid., 2.

18. Ibid.

19. Ibid.

20. Robert Browning, *The Pied Piper of Hamelin* (London: Frederick Warne and Co., 1888), 3.

21. Chester Brown. Annual Report to Ottawa, 1927/28, 3.

22. Ibid., 4.

23. Ibid., Letter to Dr. Page, Annual Report to Ottawa, 1931, 2.

24. Ibid., 4.

25. Chester Brown, letter to Dr. J.D. Page, Department of Pensions and National Health. April 5, 1932, 1.

26. John Malcolm Brinnin, *The Sway of the Grand Saloon* (New York: Delacorte Press, 1971), 430–431.

27. Ibid., 431.

28. *Victoria Daily Times*, December 6, 1944, 2.

29. *News Herald*, October 29, 1938, 18.

30. *Victoria Daily Times,* August 28, 1930, 4.

31. Ibid.

Chapter 11

1. Eli Mandel, "Estevan Saskatchewan," in Carol Gillanders, ed. *Theme and Image, Book 1* (Toronto: Copp Clark and Pittman, 1968), 46.

2. Government of Canada: Annual Departmental Reports, Vol. 3, 1936–37. Department of Pensions and National Health, 117.

3. *Daily Province*, October 29, 1938, 16.

4. Government of Canada: Annual Departmental Reports, Vol. 3, 1936–37. Department of Pensions and National Health, 127.

5. *Victoria Daily Times*, February 21, 1939, 4.

6. Ibid., 4.

7. *Daily Province*, February 28, 1939, 1.

8. Ibid.

9. Ibid.

10. *Victoria Daily Times*, October 3, 1939, 14.

11. Obituary of Dr. Theodore Bain, *British Columbia Medical Journal* 24, no. 9, 415. n.d.

12. Patrick Rowan, "The Battle to Get Rid of Irish Typhus," *Irish Medical Times*, October 28, 2009, 63.

13. Guenther Kreuger, interview with R.B. Jenkins, July 18, 1988, 9.

14. Seth Mnookin, *The Panic Virus* (New York: Simon and Shuster, 2011), 42.

15. Ibid.

16. R.B. Jenkins, "Some Findings in the Epidemic of Poliomyelitis in Alberta, 1927," *Canadian Public Health Journal* 20 no. 5 (May 1929), 219–24.

17. Ibid., 221.

18. Ibid., 220–23.

19. Guenther Kreuger, interview with R.B. Jenkins, 13.

20. Annual Reports of the Department of Health and Welfare, Ottawa, 1945–1951, 63–150.

21. *Victoria Daily Colonist*, October 5, 1947, 14.

22. Ibid., 14.

23. Guenther Kreuger, interview with R. B. Jenkins, 11.

24. *Victoria Daily Colonist*, December 22, 1954, 1.

25. Ibid.

26. Ibid.

27. *Victoria Daily Times*, September 11, 1957, 16.

28. *Victoria Daily Colonist*, August 30, 1957, 14.

29. Ibid.

30. Andrew St. Paul Butler, The History of William Head, 63.

31. Ibid.

32. Ibid., 64.

33. *Victoria Daily Times*, July 9, 1959, 17.

34. *Victoria Daily Times*, July 24, 1959, 6.

35. Ibid., 17.

36. Ibid., July 9 and 24, pp. 17 and 6 respectively.

37. *Victoria Daily Colonist*, July 25, 1959, 13.

38. Personal interview with Michael Lee, Kelowna, BC, September 12, 2010.

39. Joseph Topinka, "Yaw, Pitch and Roll: Quarantine and Isolation at United States Airports," *Public Health* 123 (March 2009), 72.

40. Personal interview with Diana Jenkins, daughter of Dr. Jenkins, April 10, 2010.

41. Ibid., 13.

42. Dr. G.M. Findlay. "Report to British Medical Journal" as reported in *Flight Magazine*. Jan. 23, 1947, 95.

Chapter 12

1. Thomas Wellems and Christopher Plowe, "Chloroquine-Resistant Malaria," *Journal of Infectious Disease* 184, no. 6 (September 2001), 770–774. This is a fine paper on the attempts by the scientific community to combat drug-resistant malaria. It's a little technical, but it shows clearly the degree to which researchers are directing their energies to probe the mechanisms of increasing drug-resistance.

2. Madeline Drexler, *Emerging Epidemics* (New York: Penguin Books, 2010), 2.

3. Wendy E. Parmet, "Stigma, Hysteria, and HIV," The Hastings Center Report 38, no. 5, 2008, 21.

4. Ibid.

5. Madeline Drexler, *Emerging Epidemics*, 276.

6. Ibid., 274.

7. Ibid., 274.

8. *Toronto Star*, December 15, 2009.

9. B. Bennett "Legal Rights during Pandemics: Federalism, Legal Rights and Public Health Laws—A View from Australia," *Public Health* 123 (March 2009), 232.

10. Maryn McKenna, "The Reason Why This Deadly E Coli Makes Doctors Shudder," *The Guardian*, June 6, 2011, 24.

11. Ibid.

12. Ibid.

13. Ibid. 14. Susan Breslowe Sardonne, *Sea-Sick: The Norwalk Virus Srikes. About.com.*, http://honeymoons.about.com/od/cruising/a/Seasick.htm.

15. Joseph B. Topinka, "Yaw, Pitch, and Roll," 52.

16. Ibid.

17. Quarantine Regulations C.R.C., c. 1368 Quarantine Act, Canadian Legal Information Institute, www.canlii.org/en/ca/laws/reg/crc-c-1368.html.

18. IATA statistics as recorded on Wikipedia.

19. Ibid.

20. Joseph Topinka, "Yaw, Pitch, and Roll," 52.

21. IATA statistics.

22. Telephone interview with Leslie Ann George and Ramon Sandhu, quarantine officers (nurses) at the Vancouver International Airport, April 25, 2010.

23. Ibid.

24. *Montreal Star*, May 25, 2007.

25. Ibid.

26. Ibid.

27. Telephone interview with Leslie Ann George and Ramon Sandhu, January 2010.

28. Air Canada pilot.

29. Personal interview with Dr. V. Montessorri, Infectious Diseases Unit, St. Paul's Hospital, Vancouver, BC, January, 2010.

30. Ibid.

31. CBC Radio News, September 14, 2011.

32. George Bush, "Quarantine May Be an Effective Response to Avian Flu," in *Pandemics*, David M. Haugen and Susan Musser, eds. (New York: Thomson Gale & Sons, 2007), 39.

33. See Wendy Orent, "Quarantine Would Not Be an Effective Response to Avian Flu," in *Pandemics*, David M. Haugen and Susan Musser, eds., 42, and "The Fear Campaign," *The Washington Post*, October 16, 2005, B01.

34. Ibid., 46.

35. Ibid., 44.

36. R. Bennett, "Legal Rights during Pandemics," 233.

Afterword

1. Louis MacNeice, "Prayer before Birth," In *Theme and Image*, Carol Gillanders, ed. (Toronto: Copp Clark Pittman, 1967), 100.

SELECTED BIBLIOGRAPHY

Newspapers

Collingwood Bulletin
Irish Medical Times
Kievlianin (Kiev Daily)
New York Times
Toronto Mail
Toronto Star
Vancouver Daily News-Advertiser
Vancouver Courier
Vancouver Province
Vancouver Sun
Victoria Daily Colonist
Victoria Daily Times
Washington Post

Magazines

The Beaver Magazine
The Islander
MacLean's Magazine
Nature
The New Yorker
Newsweek
Science
Scientific American
Time
Victoria Sunday Times Magazine

Journals

Annals of Internal Medicine
Biological Review
British Columbia Historical News
British Columbia Historical Quarterly
British Columbia Medical Association
    Journal
British Medical Journal
Bulletin of the World Health Organization
Canadian Bulletin of Medical History
Canadian Medical Association Journal
    (CMAJ)
Canadian Public Health Journal
História Ciênsias, Saúde-Manguinhos
Journal of the American Medical Association
    (JAMA)
Journal of Clinical Pharmacology and
    Therapeutics
Journal of Infection
Journal of Infectious Diseases
Journal of Legal Medicine
The Lancet
Law, Social Justice and Global Development
Medical Anthropology Quarterly
New England Journal of Medicine
Pacific Northwest Quarterly
Victoria Historical Society Publication

Articles and Books

Adler, Jerry, and Jeneen Interlandi. "Caution: Killing Germs May Be Hazardous to Your Health." *Newsweek*, October 29, 2007, 44.

Alland, Alexander. "Ecology and Adaptation to Parasitic Diseases." In *Environment and Cultural Behavior*, edited by Andrew Peter Vayda, 890–89. New York: Natural History Press, 1969.

Ambrose, Linda. "Quarantine in Question." *Canadian Bulletin of Medical History* 22, no.1 (2005): 139–53.

Armstrong, Bart. "Quarantined in Name Only: The Albert Head Story." *The Islander*, December 30, 1984, 4–5.

Arrizabulaga, John, Roger French, and John Henderson, eds. *The Great Pox*. New Haven: Yale University Press, 1997.

Basch, Paul. *Vaccines and World Health: Science, Policy, Practice*. Oxford: Oxford University Press, 1994.

Behbehani, Abbas M. "The Smallpox Story: Life and Death of an Old Disease." *Microbiological Reviews* 47, no. 4 (December 1983): 89.

Bennett, B. "Legal Rights during Pandemics: Federalism, Legal Rights and Public Health Laws—A View from Australia." *Public Health* 123 (March 2009): 232–36.

Berkelman, R.L., and J.M. Hughes. "The Conquest of Infectious Diseases: Who Are We Kidding?" *Annals of Internal Medicine* 119, no. 5 (1993): 426–28.

Bloom, B.R. "Tuberculosis: Back to a Frightening Future." *Nature* 358 (1992): 591–93

Blower, R.M., P.M. Small, and P.C. Hopewell. "Control Strategies for Tuberculosis Epidemics." *Science* 273 (1996): 497–500.

Bollet, Alfred F. *Plagues and Poxes*. New York: Demos Medical Publications, 2004.

Brinnin, John. *The Sway of the Grand Saloon*. New York: Delacorte Press, 1971.

Brown, Chester. Letter to Dr. J.D. Page, April 2, 1931. "Annual Report to Ottawa," 1931.

Butler, Alexander St. Paul. "Short History of William Head." Unpublished manuscript, Metchosin School Museum, Metchosin, British Columbia.

Cameron, Ian. *Quarantine: What Is Old Is New*. Halifax: New World Publications, 2005.

Carmichael, Mary. "Spring Fevers: Mumps Makes a Comeback in the Midwest." *Newsweek*, April 21, 2006.

Chandler, Cliff. "Chinese Labour Camps at William Head Quarantine Station, 1917–1920." *Victoria Historical Society Publication,* no. 17 (Autumn 2008): 3–4.

Davison, J. Robert. "The Chinese at William Head: A Photograph Album." *British Columbia Historical News* 16, no. 4 (1983): 18–20.

Defoe, Daniel. *A Journal of the Plague Year*. New York: Harcourt and Brace, 1985.

Dietz, Frederick. *Political and Social History of England*. New York: Macmillan Co., 1945.

Drexler, Madeline. *Secret Agents: The Menace of Emerging Infections*. Washington, DC: Joseph Henry Press, 2002.

Edelson, Paul. "Quarantine and Social Inequity." *Journal of the American Medical Association* 290, no. 21 (2003): 2874.

Esquimalt Silver Threads Writers Group. *Seafarers, Saints and Sinners: Tales of Esquimalt and Victoria West People: History and Reminiscences*. Victoria, BC: Desktop Publishing, Ltd. 1994.

Farmer, Paul. *AIDS and Accusation: Haiti and the Geography of Blame*. Berkeley: University of California Press, 1992.

———. "AIDS and Anthropologists: Ten Years Later." *Medical Anthropology Quarterly* 11, no. 4 (1997): 516–25.

———. *Infections and Inequalities: The Modern Plagues.* Berkeley: University of California Press, 1999.

Ferguson, Gerry. "Control of the Insane in British Columbia 1849–78: Care, Cure or Confinement?" In *Regulating Lives: Historical Essays on the State, Society, the Individual, and the Law,* edited by John McLaren, Robert Menzies and Dorothy E. Chunn, 63–96. Vancouver, BC: University of British Columbia Press, 2002.

Foster, G.M., and B.G. Anderson. *Medical Anthropology.* New York: Wiley & Sons, 1978.

French, Roger, ed. *Medicine from the Black Death to the French Disease.* Brookfield: Ashgate Press, 1998.

Gaudet, Marcia. *Carville: Remembering Leprosy in America.* Jackson: University Press of Mississippi, 2004.

Gilman, Ernest B. "The Art of Medicine." *The Lancet* 373, no. 9680 (June 2009): 1997–2082.

Glynn, Jennifer. *The Life and Death of Smallpox.* London: Profile Books, 2004.

Goldberg, R., S. Roach, D. Wallinga, and M. Mellon. "The Risks of Pigging Out on Antibiotics." *Science* 321 (September 2008): 1294.

Gourley, Ilma Salazar. "D'Arcy Island 1891–1907." *British Columbia Historical News* 18, no. 3 (1985).

Graham, B. *World at Risk.* New York: Vintage Books, 2008.

Gray, J.H. *The Quarantine Claims,* June 1873. British Columbia Archives HR WA 33DC 2 Q36.

Green, Valerie. *Above Stairs: Social Life in Upper Class Victoria, 1843–1918.* Victoria, BC: Sono Nis Press, 1995.

Guteri, F. "Polio's Last Stand." *Newsweek,* January 22, 2009.

Gwatkin, D.R., and P. Heuveline. "Improving the Health of the World's Poor." *British Medical Journal* 315 (1997): 497–98.

Hacking, Norman. "Ship and Shore." *Harbour and Shipping.* Vancouver, BC: Publication of *British Columbia Magazine,* 1984.

Hacking, Norman, and William Kaye Lamb. *The Princess Story.* Vancouver, BC: Mitchell Press, 1974.

Hamilton, Douglas. "The Great Pox." *Raincoast Chronicles,* no. 17 (1996).

Hansen, Helena, and Nora Groce. "Human Immunodeficiency Virus and Quarantine in Cuba." *Journal of the American Medical Association* 290, no. 21 (December 2003): 2875.

Haugen, David M., and Susan Musser, eds. *Pandemics.* New York: Thomson Gale and Sons, 2007.

Heagerty, John. *Four Centuries of Medical History in Canada.* 2 vols. Toronto: Macmillan and Co., 1928.

Helgesen, Marion. *Footprints: Pioneer Families of the Metchosin District, 1851–1900.* Metchosin, BC: Metchosin School Museum Society, 1983.

Helman, Cecil. *Culture, Health and Illness.* Bristol: Wright Press, 1984.

Hiatt, H. *Medical Lifeboat.* New York: Harper & Row, 1987.

Ho, David, D. "Time to Hit HIV, Early and Hard." *New England Journal of Medicine* 333, no. 7 (1995): 450–51.

Huntley, J. Letter to Dr. J.C. Davie, August 10, 1892. Victoria, BC: British Columbia Legislature Sessional Papers, vol. 56, 1892.

Jenkins, R.B. "Some Findings in the Epidemic of Poliomyelitis in Alberta in 1927." *Canadian Public Health Journal* 20, no. 5 (1929).

Johnson, Patricia. "McCreight and the Bench." *British Columbia Historical Quarterly* 13, no. 3 (July 1948): 211–30.

Juncosa, B. "Antibiotic Resistance: Blame It on Lifesaving Malaria Drug." *Scientific American*, July 21, 2008.

Kelly, John. *The Great Mortality. The History of the Black Death.* New York: Harper Collins, 2005.

Kilwein, J.H. "Some Historical Comments on Quarantine: Part One." *Journal of Clinical Pharmacology and Therapeutics* 20 (1995): 185–87.

Krueger, Guenther. "Interview with Dr. Roy Jenkins. Unpublished manuscript, Metchosin School Museum, Metchosin, BC.

———."The Lepers of Bentinck." *The Beaver* 69, no. 3 (1989): 60–62.

de Kruif, Paul. *Microbe Hunters.* New York: Harcourt, World and Brace, 1926.

Kuchment, Anna. "Trapping the Superbugs." *Newsweek*, December 13, 2004.

Large, R. Geddes. *Drums and Scalpel.* Vancouver, BC: Mitchell Press, 1968.

Laxton, Edward. *The Famine Ships.* London: Bloomsbury, 1966.

Lillard, Charles. *Seven Shillings a Year: The History of Vancouver Island.* Victoria, BC: Horsdal and Schubart, 1993.

Loeb, Mark, Fiona Smaill, and Mark Smieja, eds. *Evidence-Based Infectious Diseases.* Chichester, UK: BMJ/Wiley-Blackwell, 2009.

Lugrin, Nancy de Bertrand. "10,000 Coolies and a Lost Little Girl." *Victoria Sunday Times Magazine*, August 1951.

Mackie, Richard. *The Wilderness Profound.* Victoria, BC: Sono Nis Press, 1995.

Marble, Allan Everett. *Surgeons, Smallpox and the Poor.* Montreal: McGill-Queen's University Press, 1993.

Markel, Howard. *When Germs Travel.* New York: Pantheon Books, 2004.

———. *Quarantine: Jewish Immigrants in New York City during the Epidemic of 1892.* Baltimore: Johns Hopkins University Press, 1997.

Marmot, M.G. "Culture and Illness: Epidemiological Evidence." In *Foundations of Psychosomatics*, edited by M.J. Christie and P.G. Mellett, 323–40. Chichester, UK: Wiley and Sons, 1981.

Mawani, Renisa. "'The Island of the Unclean': Race, Colonialism and 'Chinese Leprosy' in British Columbia, 1891–1924." *Law, Social Justice and Global Development*, no. 1 (2003). Electronic Law Journals. http/elj.warwick.ac.uk/global/03-1/mawani.html.

McCook, James. "James Bay House of Sadness." In *Camus Chronicles of James Bay.* Victoria, BC: Camus Historical Group, 1978.

McCormick, J.B., and S.P. Fisher-Hoch. *Level 4: Virus Hunters of the CDC.* Atlanta: Turner Publishing Inc., 1996.

McCullers, J.A. "Planning for an Influenza Pandemic." *Journal of Infectious Diseases*, 198 (2008): 945–47.

McGough, Laura J. *Gender, Sexuality and Syphilis in Early Modern Venice: The Disease that Came to Stay.* London: Palgrave Macmillan, 2011.

McIntyre, John, and Stuart Houston. "Smallpox and Its Control in Canada." *Canadian Medical Association Journal* 16, no. 12 (December 1999).

McKechnie, Robert E. *Strong Medicine: History of Healing on the Northwest Coast.* Vancouver, BC: J.J. Douglas, 1972.

McKenzie, Hamish. *Infectious Diseases: Clinical Cases Uncovered.* Chichester, UK: Wiley-Blackwell, 2009.

Mnookin, Seth. *The Panic Virus.* New York: Simon and Shuster, 2011.

Moote, Lloyd, and Dorothy Moote. *The Great Plague: The Story of London's Most Deadly Year.* London and Baltimore: Johns Hopkins University Press, 2004.

Morens, David M., and Anthony S. Fauci. "The 1918 Influenza Pandemic: Insights for the 21st Century." *Journal of Infectious Diseases* 195 (April 2007): 1018–28.

Munro, A.S. "The Medical History of British Columbia." *Canadian Medical Association Journal* (September 1931): 336–42.

Novotny, Ann. *Strangers at the Door: Ellis Island, Castle Garden, and the Great Immigration to America.* Riverside, Connecticut: Chatham Press, 1971.

Orent, Wendy. "Quarantine Would Not Be an Effective Response to Avian Flu." In *Pandemics*, David M. Haugen and Susan Musser, eds. New York: Thomson Gale and Sons, 2007.

Parmet, Wendy E. "Stigma, Hysteria and HIV." *Hastings Center Report* 38, no. 5 (2008): 57.

Park, Alice. "Fighting Drug-Resistant Bugs." *Time Magazine*, June 7, 2007. http://content.time.com/time/magazine/article/0,9171,1630541,00.html.

Porter, Stephen. *The Great Plague.* Phoenix: Sutton Publications, 1990.

Puget, Peter. "Log of the Discovery, May 7–June 11, 1792." *Pacific Northwest Quarterly* 30, no. 2 (1939): 177–217.

Roizman, Bernard. *Infectious Diseases in an Age of Change.* Washington, DC: National Academic Press, 1995.

Rose, Theodore F. *From Shaman to Modern Medicine: A Century of the Healing Arts in British Columbia.* Vancouver: Mitchell Press, 1972.

Roth, J.A., C.A. Bolin, K.A. Brogden, F.C. Minion, and M.J. Wannemuehler, eds. *Virulence Mechanisms of Bacterial Pathogens.* Washington, DC: ASM Press, 1995.

Rowan, Patrick. "The Battle to Get Rid of Irish Typhus." *Irish Medical Times*, October 2009.

Santos, Fernando Sergio. "Chaulmoogra Oil as Scientific Knowledge: The Construction of a Treatment for Leprosy." *História Ciênsias, Saúde-Manguinhos* 15, no.1 (Jan/Mar 2008): 29–46.

Scheld, W. Michael, Barbara E. Murray, James M. Hughes, eds. *Emerging Infections* 6 Washington, D.C.: ASM Press, 2004.

Shepperson, W.S. *British Emigration to North America: Projects and Opinions in the Early Victorian Period.* Oxford: Basil Blackwell, 1957.

Shermin, Irwin. *Twelve Diseases that Shook the World.* Washington: American Medical Society, 2007.

Smedman, Lisa. "Coolie Express." *Vancouver Courier*, June, 26, 2009.

Specter, Michael. "Nature's Bioterrorist." *The New Yorker*, February 5, 2005.

Tanner, M., and D. de Savigny. "Malaria Eradication Back on the Table." *Bulletin of the World Health Organization* 86, no. 2 (Feb 2008): 82.

Topinka, Joseph. "Yaw, Pitch and Roll: Quarantine and Isolation at United States Airports." *Journal of Legal Medicine* 30, no. 1 (Jan–Mar 2009): 51–81.

Turner, Robert D. *The Pacific Empresses*. Victoria: Sono Nis Press, 1981.

Vancouver, George. *The Voyage of Discovery to the North Pacific and Round the World*. London: G. Robinson and Co., 1798.

Walker, George Alfred. *Burial Ground Incendiarism*. London: Longman and Co., 1845.

Walsh, Bryan. "Danger from the Bird-Flu Drug." *Time.com*, March 20, 2007. http://content.time.com/time/health/article/0,8599,1601062,00.html.

Wang, H., Z. Feng, S. Yuelong, et al. "Probable Limited Person-to-Person Transmission of Highly Pathogenic Avian Influenza A (H5N1) Virus in China." *The Lancet* 371, no. 9622 (2008): 1427–34.

Waring, R.H., G.B. Steventon, S.C. Mitchell, eds. *Molecules of Death*. London: Imperial College Press, 2007.

Wellems, Thomas, and Chris Plowe. "Chloroquine-Resistant Malaria." *The Journal of Infectious Disease* 184, no. 6 (September 2001): 770–76.

Wickberg, Edgar, ed. *From China to Canada: A History of Chinese Communities in Canada*. Toronto: McClelland & Stewart, 1988.

Wills, Christopher. *Yellow Fever, Black Goddess: The Co-evolution of People and Plagues*. Reading, Massachusetts: Helix Books, 1996.

Yortath, Chris. *A Measure of Value: The Story of D'Arcy Island*. Victoria, BC: Touchwood Publications, 2000.

Young, Cy. "Lepers' Island." *MacLean's Magazine*, May 1, 1948.

INDEX

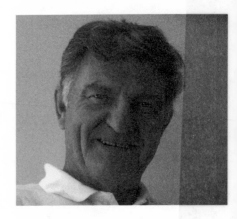

Peter Johnson has taught history, English, and creative writing in high schools and colleges in Canada for over thirty-five years. He has written two previous books, *Glyphs and Gallows: The Rock Art of Clo-oose and the Wreck of the John Bright* and *Voyages of Hope: The Saga of the Brideships*. He has also written and directed a documentary film on Lake Winnipeg, which was shown on CBC television, and published interpretive articles on Dostoevsky's *The Brothers Karamazov* and George Orwell's *1984*. He lives in Vancouver, British Columbia.